Handbook of Integrative Oncology Nursing: Evidence-Based Practice

by
Georgia M. Decker, APRN, ANP-BC, CN®, CLNC, AOCN®
CDR Colleen O. Lee, MS, CRNP, CLNC, AOCN®

Guest Contributor
Linda U. Krebs, RN, PhD, AOCN®, FAAN

D1373850

Oncology Nursing Society
Pittsburgh, PA

ONS Publishing Division
Publisher: Leonard Mafrica, MBA, CAE
Director of Publications: Barbara Sigler, RN, MNEd
Managing Editor: Lisa M. George, BA
Technical Content Editor: Angela D. Klimaszewski, RN, MSN
Staff Editor: Amy Nicoletti, BA
Copy Editor: Laura Pinchot, BA
Graphic Designer: Dany Sjoen

Cover photo courtesy of Colleen Lee; photo taken at Glenmont Park in Silver Spring, Maryland, May 2009.

Library of Congress Cataloging-in-Publication Data
Decker, Georgia M.
  Handbook of integrative oncology nursing : evidence-based practice / by Georgia M. Decker and Colleen O. Lee.
    p. ; cm.
  Includes bibliographical references and index.
  ISBN 978-1-890504-94-6 (alk. paper)
  1. Cancer–Nursing. 2. Cancer–Alternative treatment. 3. Evidence-based nursing. I. Lee, Colleen O. II. Oncology Nursing Society. III. Title.
  [DNLM: 1. Neoplasms–nursing. 2. Complementary Therapies–nursing. 3. Evidence-Based Nursing. WY 156 D295h 2010]
  RC266.D42 2010
  616.99'40231–dc22

                                                                                        2010016224

Publisher's Note
    This book is published by the Oncology Nursing Society (ONS). ONS neither represents nor guarantees that the practices described herein will, if followed, ensure safe and effective patient care. The recommendations contained in this book reflect ONS's judgment regarding the state of general knowledge and practice in the field as of the date of publication. The recommendations may not be appropriate for use in all circumstances. Those who use this book should make their own determinations regarding specific safe and appropriate patient-care practices, taking into account the personnel, equipment, and practices available at the hospital or other facility at which they are located. The editors and publisher cannot be held responsible for any liability incurred as a consequence from the use or application of any of the contents of this book. Figures and tables are used as examples only. They are not meant to be all-inclusive, nor do they represent endorsement of any particular institution by ONS. Mention of specific products and opinions related to those products do not indicate or imply endorsement by ONS. Web sites mentioned are provided for information only; the hosts are responsible for their own content and availability. Unless otherwise indicated, dollar amounts reflect U.S. dollars.
    ONS publications are originally published in English. Publishers wishing to translate ONS publications must contact the ONS Publishing Division about licensing arrangements. ONS publications cannot be translated without obtaining written permission from ONS. (Individual tables and figures that are reprinted or adapted require additional permission from the original source.) Because translations from English may not always be accurate or precise, ONS disclaims any responsibility for inaccuracies in words or meaning that may occur as a result of the translation. Readers relying on precise information should check the original English version.

Printed in the United States of America

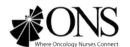

Oncology Nursing Society

Integrity • Innovation • Stewardship • Advocacy • Excellence • Inclusiveness

To our colleagues and patients, you continue to inspire us daily as we work together to build the bridge to integrative oncology care.

Disclosure

Editors and authors of books and guidelines provided by the Oncology Nursing Society are expected to disclose to the participants any significant financial interest or other relationships with the manufacturer(s) of any commercial products.

A vested interest may be considered to exist if a contributor is affiliated with or has a financial interest in commercial organizations that may have a direct or indirect interest in the subject matter. A "financial interest" may include, but is not limited to, being a shareholder in the organization; being an employee of the commercial organization; serving on an organization's speakers bureau; or receiving research from the organization. An "affiliation" may be holding a position on an advisory board or some other role of benefit to the commercial organization. Vested interest statements appear in the front matter for each publication.

Contributors are expected to disclose any unlabeled or investigational use of products discussed in their content. This information is acknowledged solely for the information of the readers.

The contributors provided the following disclosure and vested interest information:

The authors have no relevant information to disclose.

Contents

Introduction

Defining Complementary and Alternative Medicine

Throughout this handbook, the acronym *CAM* refers to complementary and alternative medicine therapies, and the term *conventional* refers to traditional or standard approaches. Conventional approaches are those that historically have broad application in Western medicine (National Center for Complementary and Alternative Medicine [NCCAM], 2009). CAM therapies also are termed *integrative, integrated,* or *complementary* when these therapies are combined with conventional approaches. The term *alternative* refers to a CAM therapy that is used *instead of* a conventional treatment. The intention with which a therapy is used best describes it. The interchangeable use of these terms can cause miscommunication and misunderstanding between patients and healthcare professionals (HCPs), as well as among HCPs (Decker & Lee, 2005). Additional terminology is explained in Appendix I.

Whorton (1999) suggested that an awareness of the historical development of CAM is essential to understand the philosophical viewpoints among practitioners through the years to the present. Prior to the 19th century, unconventional methods of disease treatment were considered folk medicine or quackery. The second generation of developing medical systems began in the late 20th century and was represented within osteopathy, chiropractic, naturopathy, and hydropathy. Simultaneously, contemporary holism emerged, focusing on treating the "whole" patient. This led to the current movement of wellness promotion (Gallin, 2002). During the 1950s, nursing curricula made a distinction between patient needs and problems from a medical diagnosis (Black & Matassarin-Jacobs, 1993).

Contemporary Complementary and Alternative Medicine Use

Consumers continued to seek CAM therapies despite the medical advances of the 1970s and 1980s. Because of increasing significant issues within the field, the Office of Alternative Medicine (OAM) was established in 1992. In 1998, OAM became NCCAM. To increase high-quality research and information about CAM use specifically within the oncology population, the National Cancer Institute (NCI) established the Office of Cancer Complementary and Alternative Medicine (OCCAM) in 1998 as well. OCCAM is responsible for NCI's resource agenda in CAM as it related to cancer prevention, diagnosis, treatment, and symptom management. In March 2000, the White House Commission on Complementary and Alternative Medicine Policy (2002) convened to further address significant issues such as access to and delivery of CAM, research priorities, and consumer and HCP education. In 2003–2004, the Institute of Medicine (IOM) of the National Academies, a non-government agency established in 1970, sponsored seven committee meetings to investigate scientific, policy, and practice questions that arise from the increasing use of CAM. IOM guarantees unbiased, evidence-based information and advice concerning health and science policy to policy makers, HCPs, and the public (IOM, 2004).

Surveys of Complementary and Alternative Medicine Use

Early surveys of CAM use were not population or diagnosis specific (Eisenberg et al., 1993; Ernst & Cassileth, 1998). However, by the beginning of 2000, researchers had accumulated sufficient amount of publishable data regarding CAM use in the oncology population (Ashikaga, Bosompra, O'Brien, & Nelson, 2002; Nam, Fleshner, & Rakovitch, 1999; Swisher et al., 2002). When compared with non-CAM users, individuals who use CAM are more likely to be female, better educated, and have higher incomes (Ernst & Cassileth; IOM, 2004; Sparber et al., 2000). Although the quality and quantity of information about CAM use have increased, much remains to be learned about specific indications and contraindications for specific therapies when used in specific clinical situations, as well as clarification of the role and scope of HCPs in CAM. Contemporary efforts speak to this clarification within professional societies and academic settings.

Guidelines for Complementary and Alternative Medicine Use

Formalized guidelines for CAM use were not in existence until recently. Theoretically, documents of this type offer a foundation for societal, academic, consumer, and healthcare approaches to CAM use. Examples are (a) Society for Integrative Oncology's *Evidence-Based Clinical Practice Guidelines for Integrative Oncology* (see Appendix II) and (b) American Cancer Society's (ACS's)

Guidelines for Using Complementary and Alternative Methods (ACS, 2009). They lack, however, recognition and acknowledgment of the fundamental role of nursing in integrative oncology. The position statement of the American Holistic Nurses Association (AHNA) directly addresses the nurse's role in the practice of complementary and alternative therapies (AHNA, 2008). To recognize the fundamental role of nursing in cancer care, the Oncology Nursing Society (ONS, 2008) offered its position statement, *The Use of Complementary and Alternative Therapies in Cancer Care* (see Appendix III).

Integrative Oncology Nursing Role

Lee (2003, 2004) offered that oncology nurses must become knowledgeable in integrative oncology given the rapidly increasing use of CAM. The model for integrative oncology nursing care begins with the nurse, the patient, and other healthcare team members and endorses three core actions: (a) distinguishing fact from fiction, (b) acknowledging misperceptions about CAM, and (c) mixing and un-mixing therapies. End points for nursing are as follows (Lee, 2004):

- Expand individual baseline knowledge regarding cancer CAM through oral and written modes with experiential learning.
- Provide high-quality patient and peer education regarding safety and efficacy of CAM therapies.
- Facilitate partnerships between patients, conventional HCPs, CAM providers, and colleagues to discuss knowledge and perspectives about cancer CAM.
- Seek proper training, demonstrate competency, and obtain necessary credentials if practicing a CAM therapy.
- Request and require informed consent (with witness) of patients receiving a CAM therapy.
- Ensure proper credentialing of a CAM provider prior to recommending the provider to patients.
- Establish institutional-specific standards of practice for the use of CAM therapies within specific patient populations.
- Document patient consent procedures, tolerance, and response to CAM therapy.
- Design a new program or assist in the quality maintenance of a pre-established integrative care program.
- Develop and update a working knowledge of cost issues and reimbursement of CAM in the community.
- Collaborate in the design of methodologically rigorous cancer CAM treatment and supportive care clinical trials.
- Contribute to the body of nursing knowledge in cancer CAM through publications and presentations in the United States and internationally.

The future holds opportunities for nursing to demonstrate and claim a fundamental role in integrative oncology. This begins with the expansion of nurses' knowledge of CAM. The goal of this handbook is to promote evidence-based practice within integrative oncology nursing by synthesizing present knowledge with regard to safety, efficacy, concurrent use with conventional therapy, and long-term use across the cancer continuum.

References

American Cancer Society. (2009). *Guidelines for using complementary and alternative methods.* Retrieved August 24, 2009, from http://www.cancer.org/docroot/ETO/content/ETO_5_3x_Guidelines_For_Using_Complementary_and_Alternative_Methods.asp

American Holistic Nurses Association. (2008). *Position on the role of nurses in the practice of complementary and alternative therapies.* Retrieved August 20, 2009, from http://www.ahna.org/Resources/Publications/PositionStatements/tabid/1926/Default.aspx

Ashikaga, T., Bosompra, K., O'Brien, P., & Nelson, L. (2002). Use of complementary and alternative medicine by breast cancer patients: Prevalence, patterns and communication with physicians. *Supportive Care in Cancer, 10*(7), 542–548.

Black. J.M., & Matassarin-Jacobs, E. (1993). Nursing process. In J.M. Black & E. Matassarin-Jacobs (Eds.), *Luckmann and Sorensen's medical-surgical nursing: A psychophysiologic approach* (4th ed., pp. 1–2). Philadelphia: W.B. Saunders.

Decker, G., & Lee, C.O. (2005). Complementary and alternative medicine (CAM) therapies. In C.H. Yarbro, M.H. Frogge, & M. Goodman (Eds.), *Cancer nursing: Principles and practice* (6th ed., pp. 590–620). Sudbury, MA: Jones and Bartlett.

Eisenberg, D.M., Kessler, R.C., Foster, C., Norlock, F.E., Calkins, D.R., & Delbanco, T.L. (1993). Unconventional medicine in the United States. Prevalence, costs, and patterns of use. *New England Journal of Medicine, 328*(4), 246–252.

Ernst, E., & Cassileth, B.R. (1998). The prevalence of complementary/alternative medicine in cancer: A systematic review. *Cancer, 83*(4), 777–782.

Gallin, J.I. (2002). A historical perspective on clinical research. In J.I. Gallin (Ed.), *Principles and practice of clinical research* (pp. 1–11). San Diego, CA: Academic Press.

Institute of Medicine of the National Academies. (2004). *Use of complementary and alternative (CAM) therapies by the American public.* Washington, DC: Author.

Lee, C.O. (2003, November). *CAM in the 21st century in the US: Role of nursing and evidence-based practice efforts.* Poster session presented at the 4th Annual Oncology Nursing Society Institutes of Learning, Philadelphia, PA.

Lee, C.O. (2004). Clinical trials in cancer part II. Biomedical, complementary, and alternative medicine: Significant issues. *Clinical Journal of Oncology Nursing, 8*(6), 670–674.

Nam, R.K., Fleshner, N., & Rakovitch, E. (1999). Prevalence and patterns of the use of complementary therapies among prostate cancer patients: An epidemiological analysis. *Journal of Urology, 161*(5), 1521–1524.

National Center for Complementary and Alternative Medicine. (2009). *What is complementary and alternative medicine?* Retrieved August 26, 2009, from http://nccam.nih.gov/health/whatiscam/

Oncology Nursing Society. (2008). *The use of complementary and alternative therapies in cancer care.* Retrieved November 12, 2009, from http://www.ons.org/Publications/Positions/media/ons/docs/positions/alternativetherapies.pdf

Sparber, A., Bauer, L., Curt, G., Eisenberg, D., Levin, T., Parks, S., et al. (2000). Use of complementary medicine by adult patients participating in cancer clinical trials. *Oncology Nursing Forum, 27*(4), 623–630.

Swisher, E.M., Cohn, D.E., Goff, B.A., Parham, J., Herzog, T.J., Rader, J.S., et al. (2002). Use of complementary and alternative medicine among women with gynecologic cancers. *Gynecologic Oncology, 84*(3), 363–367.

White House Commission on Complementary and Alternative Medicine Policy. (2002). *Final report.* Washington, DC: U.S. Department of Health and Human Services. Retrieved December 21, 2009, from http://govinfo.library.unt.edu/whccamp/pdfs/fr2002_document.pdf

Whorton, J.C. (1999). The history of complementary and alternative medicine. In W.B. Jonas & J.S. Levin (Eds.), *Essentials of complementary and alternative medicine* (pp. 16–30). Philadelphia: Lippincott Williams & Wilkins.

The Integrative Assessment: A Cornerstone for Integrative Oncology Nursing

An integrated assessment conducted by HCPs identifies information that is applicable regarding past and current use of CAM for comorbidities and cancer- and cancer treatment–related symptoms in addition to traditional assessment. Health professionals must communicate a willingness to understand the value and significance of CAM to patients in order to conduct a meaningful integrative assessment. Creating a nonjudgmental environment that allows patients to express their willingness and desire to be a partner in decisions regarding their care is vital to the integrative assessment. Decker (2005) offered an algorithm to assist HCPs in communicating with patients about CAM (see Figure 1).

Although no single integrative assessment tool has been nationally vetted, thought leaders agree on core components (Jonas, Linde, & Walach, 1999; Lee, 2009; Maizes, Koffler, & Fleishman, 2002):

- Health history basics: Demographics (including insurance), chief complaint, history of present illness, past medical history, medications (including adherence), allergies, social history, immunizations and travel, family history, review of systems, laboratory tests, diagnostics
- Integrative assessment basics: Comprehensive medication assessment, previous and current CAM therapies (including use, duration, reason, benefit, provider, cost, location, side effects), general well-being, nutrition, physical activity and exercise, stress management, spirituality, personal image, view toward illness state and recommended conventional therapies, and anticipated CAM use (or desire for more information)
- Treatment plan basics: Is a safe and effective conventional therapy available? Is receiving a conventional therapy desirable to the patient? Is a safe and effective CAM therapy available? Is the population studied similar to the patient? Is there a strong belief or agreement in the rationale of the CAM therapy between the HCP and patient? Is the cost of CAM therapy low?
- Can the patient be monitored during the treatment period? Is there a risk of interactions between the conventional and CAM therapies? Is a plan for consistent follow-up in place?

Integrated assessment models that can meet the needs of oncology HCPs and patients in a variety of practice settings are offered as follows. It has been suggested that organizations, institutions, and private practices have assessment forms that are compliant with federal (Medicare), state, and third-party payer requirements. A change to these forms may not be in anyone's best interest. Therefore, two models are provided: one that is inclusive of Medicare requirements and thereby meets the state requirements as well as third-party payer requirements (see Figure 2) and a shorter version that, when used with an established assessment, will create a fully integrated assessment (see Figure 3).

Figure 1. Discussing CAM Therapies With Patients

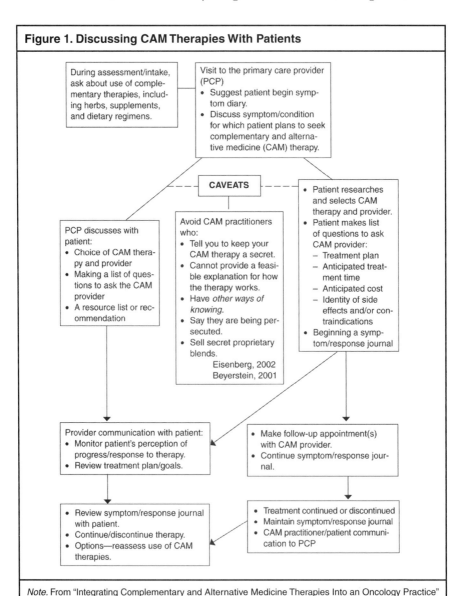

Note. From "Integrating Complementary and Alternative Medicine Therapies Into an Oncology Practice" (p. 365), by G. Decker in P.C. Buchsel and C.H. Yarbro (Eds.), *Oncology Nursing in the Ambulatory Setting: Issues and Models of Care* (2nd ed.), 2005, Sudbury, MA: Jones and Bartlett. Copyright 2005 by Jones and Bartlett. www.jbpub.com. Reprinted with permission.

Figure 2. Full Integrative Assessment

Integrative Assessment (FULL)		Date of Service:	
Name:		☐ M ☐ F	DOB:
1°Insurance Provider:		2°Insurance Provider:	

The main reason for your appointment today:

For Office Use Only:

Height:	Weight:	Usual Weight:		Pain (0–10):
T:	P:	B/P:	R:	Pulse Ox:

Current Medical Issues (Please include symptoms.)

Medical Issue or Concern	When Did It Begin?	Symptom(s):

Females, please record the first date of your last menstrual period:

Past Medical History (Please include any surgeries and recent trauma/accidents.)

Medical Condition or Surgery	When Diagnosed?	Treatment/Name of Provider

Significant Family Medical History (Please include parents and maternal and paternal grandparents.)

Who/Medical Condition or Surgery	When Diagnosed?	Treatment Received

(Continued on next page)

Figure 2. Full Integrative Assessment *(Continued)*

Allergies (Please include allergies to medicine, the environment, and food sensitivities.)

Medication Allergy	Environmental Allergy	Food Sensitivity

Ethnicity:

☐ Caucasian (specify)	☐ African American (specify)	☐ Hispanic/Latino (specify)
☐ Native American (specify tribe)		☐ Pacific Islander (specify)

Other Information:

Education

☐ Elementary	☐ Secondary	☐ Post-Secondary (specify)

☐ I smoke cigars and/or cigarettes (please specify length of time)

☐ I drink alcohol (please specify type of alcohol and number of drinks per week)

Are you in a monogamous relationship? ☐ Yes   ☐ No ☐ N/A

Medications:
Please list your current prescription and nonprescription medicines (examples follow):
Please continue information on the back of this page should you need additional space.

Prescription Medications: ear or eye drops, injectable medications (e.g., syringe, ambulatory pump, recent vaccines, anergy panels, immunizations, allergy testing), IV medications (continuous infusion and intermittent), medicated patches, medications via jejunostomy, gastrostomy, or nasogastric tube), nasal sprays and inhalation preparations (e.g., aerosols, inhalers, mist tent), oral medications (e.g., tablets, capsules, liquids, lozenges, sublingual medications), prescribed marijuana (inhalation form), rectal or vaginal suppositories or enemas, topical creams, lotions, ointments, or powders.

Nonprescription Medications: alcoholic beverages, antacids, cold and flu remedies, ear or eye drops, essential oils (applied topically or via aromatherapy), fluid products (water or juice with additives, iced or hot teas [single or combination herbs and how they are dispensed]) and drinks made in blenders, food supplement bars (containing soy, vitamins, and minerals), herbs (single or combination products), home remedies (e.g., tonics, homeopathic products), medicated patches, medications given via jejunostomy, gastrostomy, or nasogastric tube, minerals (single or combination products), nasal sprays and inhalation preparations (e.g., aerosols, inhalers, mist tent), pain relievers, rectal or vaginal suppositories or enemas, stimulants, laxatives, and antidiarrheals, tobacco products (e.g., cigars, cigarettes, chew, betel nut), topical creams, lotions, ointments, or powders, vitamins (single or combination products).

(Continued on next page)

Figure 2. Full Integrative Assessment *(Continued)*

Prescription and Nonprescription Medication	Who Prescribed or Recommended It	Dose/ Frequency	Reason(s) Why You Are Taking It

Nutrition: What do you typically eat for breakfast, lunch, dinner, and snacks?

Are you now receiving or have you ever received or participated in (please check all that apply)**:**

☐ Acupuncture	☐ Aromatherapy	☐ Art, Music, or Dance Therapy
☐ Chiropractic Therapy	☐ Counseling	☐ Supervised Exercise Program
☐ Massage	☐ Naturopathic Medicine	☐ Qigong or Tai Chi
☐ Reiki	☐ Therapeutic/Healing Touch	☐ Yoga

☐ Other

Please describe the therapy, provider/location, length of therapy, and experienced benefits or side effects:

Therapy	Provider/ Location	Length of Therapy	Benefits Experienced	Side Effects Experienced

What do you enjoy doing for relaxation and fun?

How may we help you **today**?

What information would you want to receive today?

A comprehensive guide to decision making in integrative oncology for nurses has not yet been developed. Nurses and other HCPs who are conducting these assessments are in a position to identify the practice issues related to care of patients with cancer who use CAM therapies. These issues include referral versus recommendation to CAM practitioners, billing issues, appropriate follow-up and communication with CAM practitioner, documentation challenges, and legal and ethical implications.

Figure 3. Abbreviated Integrative Assessment

Abbreviated Integrative Assessment (INITIAL AND PERMANENT EXAMINATION)	Date of Service	
Name:	☐ M ☐ F	**DOB:**
1°Insurance Provider:	**2°Insurance Provider:**	

The main reason for your appointment today:

Prescription and Nonprescription Medication	Who Prescribed or Recommended It	Dose/ Frequency	Reason(s) Why You Are Taking It

Nutrition: What do you typically eat for breakfast, lunch, dinner, and snacks?

Are you now receiving or have you ever received or participated in (please check all that apply):

☐ Acupuncture	☐ Aromatherapy	☐ Art, Music, or Dance Therapy
☐ Chiropractic Therapy	☐ Counseling	☐ Supervised Exercise Program
☐ Massage	☐ Naturopathic Medicine	☐ Qigong or Tai Chi
☐ Reiki	☐ Therapeutic/Healing Touch	☐ Yoga
☐ Other		

Please describe the therapy, provider/location, length of therapy, and experienced benefits or side effects:

Therapy	Provider/ Location	Length of Therapy	Benefits Experienced	Side Effects Experienced

(Continued on next page)

Figure 3. Abbreviated Integrative Assessment *(Continued)*
What do you enjoy doing for relaxation and fun?
How may we help you **today**?
What information would you want to receive today?
A comprehensive guide to decision making in integrative oncology for nurses has not yet been developed. Nurses and other HCPs who are conducting these assessments are in a position to identify the practice issues related to care of patients with cancer who use CAM therapies. These issues include referral versus recommendation to CAM practitioners, billing issues, appropriate follow-up and communication with CAM practitioner, documentation challenges, and legal and ethical implications.

References

Beyerstein, B.L. (2001). Alternative medicine and common errors of reasoning. *Academic Medicine, 76*(3), 230–237.

Decker, G.M. (2005). Integrating complementary and alternative medicine therapies into an oncology practice: A short history of medicine. In P.C. Buchsel & C.H. Yarbro (Eds.), *Oncology nursing in the ambulatory setting: Issues and models of care* (2nd ed., pp. 355–375). Sudbury, MA: Jones and Bartlett.

Eisenberg, D.M. (2002, March). *Complementary and integrative medicine state of the science and clinical applications.* Syllabus presented at the Complementary and Integrative Medicine: Clinical Update and Implications for Practice conference. Harvard Medical School, Department of Continuing Education, Boston, MA.

Jonas, W.B., Linde, K., & Walach, H. (1999). How to practice evidence-based complementary and alternative medicine. In W.B. Jonas & J.S. Levin (Eds.), *Essentials of complementary and alternative medicine* (pp. 72–87). Philadelphia: Lippincott Williams & Wilkins.

Lee, C.O. (2009). Complementary and integrative therapies. In B.H. Gobel, S. Triest-Robertson, & W.H. Vogel (Eds.), *Advanced oncology nursing certification review and resource manual* (pp. 305–327). Pittsburgh, PA: Oncology Nursing Society.

Maizes, V., Koffler, K., & Fleishman, S. (2002). Revisiting the health history: An integrative medicine approach. *Advances in Mind-Body Medicine, 18*(2), 31–34.

Defining and Describing Commonly Used CAM Therapies

Categorizing CAM Therapies

Two central approaches to categorizing CAM therapies exist and are widely accepted. NCCAM classifies CAM therapies into five domains: alternative medical systems, mind-body interventions, biologically based therapies, manipulative and body-based methods, and energy therapies (NCCAM, 2007). NCI OCCAM (2009) expanded the NCCAM domains with three additional categories: nutritional therapeutics, pharmacologic and biologic treatments (with subcategory of complex natural products), and spiritual therapies. In this text, the NCI OCCAM classification is used (see Table 1).

Licensure of CAM Practitioners

A CAM practitioner is normally thought to be an individual who delivers CAM therapies as a portion of his or her practice and may possess certification or licensure from a state, national, or professionally recognized program (Lee, 2009). Professional differences exist between credentialing and licensure of providers (Oliver, 2003). Licensure refers to the laws that regulate a given occupation and has two purposes: (a) to protect the title, thereby preventing unqualified practitioners from using the title, and (b) to define the scope of practice in outlining specific tasks that form the practice. Licensure occurs at the state level, and the scope of practice may vary from state to state. In most states, CAM providers who lack licensure could be viewed as diagnosing and treating patients and as practicing medicine unlawfully.

Certification of CAM Practitioners

Certification is a process in which an accrediting body grants recognition to a practitioner for meeting predetermined qualifications (e.g., didactic learning, practice hours, examination). National certification en-

Table 1. Categories of Complementary and Alternative Medicine Therapies

Domain	Description	Examples
Alternative medical systems	Systems built upon well-developed systems of theory and practice	Traditional Chinese medicine, acupuncture, Ayurveda, homeopathy, naturopathy, Tibetan medicine
Energy therapies	Therapies involving the use of energy fields	Qigong, Reiki, therapeutic touch, pulsed fields, magnet therapy
Exercise therapies	Therapies used to improve patterns of bodily movement	Tai chi, Hatha yoga, Alexander Technique, dance therapy, Rolfing®, Trager Method, applied kinesiology, Feldenkrais
Manipulative and body-based methods	Therapies based on manipulation and movement of one or more body parts	Chiropractic, massage, osteopathy, reflexology
Mind-body interventions	Therapies designed to enhance the mind's capacity to have an effect on bodily function and symptoms	Meditation, art therapy, imagery, relaxation therapy, support groups, music therapy, cognitive-behavioral therapy, aromatherapy, animal-assisted therapy
Nutritional therapeutics	Assortment of nutrients, non-nutrients, bioactive food components, and diets that are used as chemopreventive and treatment agents	Macrobiotics, vegetarianism, Gerson therapy, Kelley-Gonzalez regimen, vitamins, antioxidants, melatonin, selenium, coenzyme Q10
Pharmacologic and biologic treatments	Drugs, complex natural products, vaccines, and other biologic interventions that are not yet accepted into conventional medicine and the off-label use of prescription drugs	Antineoplastons, products from honey bees, mistletoe, 714-X, low-dose naltrexone, immuno-augmentative therapy, laetrile, hydrazine sulfate, New Castle virus, melatonin, enzyme therapy, high-dose vitamin C
Complex natural products subcategory of pharmacologic and biologic treatments	Assortment of botanicals, extracts of crude natural substances, and unfractionated extracts from marine organisms used for healing and treatment of disease	Botanicals, herbs, and herbal extracts, mixtures of tea polyphenols, shark cartilage
Spiritual therapies	Therapies focusing on religious beliefs and feelings, including an individual's sense of peace, purpose, connection with others, and beliefs about the meaning of life	Intercessory prayer, spiritual healing

Note. Based on information from National Cancer Institute Office of Cancer Complementary and Alternative Medicine, 2009; National Institutes of Health National Center for Complementary and Alternative Medicine, 2007.

sures that a professional's credentials will be recognized in all states and that the scope of practice is the same. Examples of CAM practices with educational preparation, licensure, and credentialing criteria are listed in Table 2.

Specifically for nurses, the American Holistic Nurses' Certification Corporation (www.ahncc.org) is the sole nursing body that offers an inclusive certification. Many nurses choose to undergo training in specific areas of CAM such as Reiki, bodywork, aromatherapy, or homeopathy.

Efficacy and Safety of CAM Therapies

Limited and often incomplete data exist on the safety, efficacy, and mechanism of action of many CAM therapies. Until recently, theoretical or personal opinion superseded data simply because of the lack of available evidence. The concept of an evidence-based approach to CAM remains in its infancy. Recommending CAM therapies remains challenging for HCPs as patients continue to request reliable information. This effort may intensify when conventional therapies to prevent and treat cancer and cancer-related symptoms and side effects are not providing the desired result.

Levels of Evidence in CAM

Levels of evidence and evidence-based practice in CAM are created in the same method as those in conventional medicine. Angel and Kassirer (1998) emphasized that one category of medicine exists: one that has been tested effectively, reasoning that once a therapy has been tested, it no longer matters whether it was conventional or alternative at the beginning. They affirmed that if the therapy is established as safe and effective, it can be integrated into clinical practice, but theories and testimonials do not replace evidence.

The strength of study design, strength of end points measured, and individually assessed levels of evidence scores constitute the major criteria for grading the strength and quality of conventional and CAM research. In this handbook, three reputable sources for information are used to grade available evidence in support of or not in support of a CAM therapy for cancer-related side effects and symptoms: Natural Standard, Natural Medicines Comprehensive Database, and NCI's Physician Data Query (PDQ®). Comparisons between these grading systems are seen in Table 3 with examples of the modalities in Table 4.

Table 2. Examples* of CAM Practices With Educational Preparation, Licensure, and Credentialing Criteria

Practice	Acronym	Certification or Licensing Body	Educational Preparation	Related Links
Acupuncture	LAc (licensed acupuncturist)	National Certification Commission for Acupuncture and Oriental Medicine (NCCAOM) training, licensing, and certification	NCCAOM certification is the only nationally recognized certification available to practitioners of acupuncture and Oriental medicine. NCCAOM certification is a requirement for licensure in most states.	NCCAOM www.nccaom.org
Animal-assisted activity (AAA) or animal-assisted therapy (AAT)	None specified	No formal credentialing or licensure process; many trained therapists (e.g., physical, occupational) can incorporate AAA or AAT into their practice.	The Delta Society offers a comprehensive service dog trainer curriculum according to their *Standards of Practice in Animal-Assisted Activities and Animal-Assisted Therapy.*	Delta Society www.deltasociety.org
Aromatherapy	RA (registered aromatherapist)	No formal credentialing or licensure process. Many trained practitioners incorporate essential oils into their practice.	The National Association for Holistic Aromatherapy (NAHA) approves aromatherapy courses according to their education standards. The Aromatherapy Registration Council Examination in Aromatherapy is open to anyone who has completed a minimum of a one-year level 2 program in aromatherapy from an NAHA-compliant college or school or anyone who could provide evidence of equivalent training.	NAHA www.naha.org Aromatherapy Registration Council www.aromatherapycouncil.org/index.html

(Continued on next page)

Table 2. Examples* of CAM Practices With Educational Preparation, Licensure, and Credentialing Criteria *(Continued)*

Practice	Acronym	Certification or Licensing Body	Educational Preparation	Related Links
Art therapy	ATR-BC (art therapist, board certified)	Certification is offered through the Art Therapy Credentials Board. No formal licensure process exists. Many trained practitioners incorporate art therapy into their practice.	Minimum educational and professional standards are established by the American Art Therapy Association, Inc., a membership and advocacy organization.	Art Therapy Credentials Board, Inc. www.atcb.org
Ayurveda	BAMS (bachelor of Ayurvedic medicine and surgery) DAMS (doctor of Ayurvedic medicine and surgery)	No formal licensure or certification process exists in the United States. Many trained practitioners incorporate Ayurvedic medicine into their practice.	Ayurvedic training in India is obtained with either a bachelor's degree or doctorate degree. Several states in the United States have approved Ayurvedic schools encouraging up to 500 hours of clinical practice.	National Ayurvedic Medical Association www.ayurveda-nama.org/index.php
Chiropractic medicine	DC (doctor of chiropractic medicine)	Licensure in 50 states and in Washington, DC, following a national board examination	The curriculum includes a minimum of 4,200 hours of classroom, laboratory, and clinical experience.	The American Chiropractic Association www.amerchiro.org
Healing touch	CHTP (certified healing touch practitioner)	Certification is offered through Healing Touch International, Inc. No formal licensure process is available. Many trained practitioners incorporate healing touch into their practice.	The Healing Touch Certificate Program is a continuing education program endorsed by the American Holistic Nurses Association. It is sequenced through six levels of didactic and experiential learning.	Healing Touch International, Inc. www.healingtouchinternational.org/index.php

(Continued on next page)

Table 2. Examples* of CAM Practices With Educational Preparation, Licensure, and Credentialing Criteria *(Continued)*

Practice	Acronym	Certification or Licensing Body	Educational Preparation	Related Links
Homeopathy	Hom (homeopathic physician)	A diploma or certification of completion can be obtained. No formal licensure process is available. Many trained practitioners incorporate homeopathy into their practice.	Several homeopathic programs in the United States offer a range of 10-week to 3-year curriculums In 2011, the Doctor of Classical Homeopathy Program through the American Medical College of Homeopathy will begin a full-time program, spanning four years and 4,280 clinical hours	American Medical College of Homeopathy www.amcofh.org
Macrobiotics	None at this time	No formal credentialing or licensure process is available. Certification is offered through Macrobiotics America. Many trained practitioners incorporate macrobiotics into their practice.	Several macrobiotic training programs in the United States involve online study and in-person training. Certification requires six months of learning with focus on caregiver cooking, healthy lifestyle cooking, or cooking teacher.	Macrobiotics America www.macroamerica.com/cooktraining.php The Kushi Institute www.kushiinstitute.org
Massage therapy	CMT-BC (certified massage therapist, board certified)	Certification is offered through the National Certification Board for Therapeutic Massage and Bodywork (NCBTMB) 33 states and Washington, DC, recognize NCBTMB certification.	Certification requires about 500 hours of instruction; therapist must demonstrate mastery of core skills and pass a standardized NCBTMB examination. NCBTMB programs are accredited by the National Commission for Certifying Agencies.	NCBTMB www.ncbtmb.org

(Continued on next page)

Table 2. Examples* of CAM Practices With Educational Preparation, Licensure, and Credentialing Criteria (Continued)

Practice	Acronym	Certification or Licensing Body	Educational Preparation	Related Links
Music therapy	MT-BC (music therapist, board certified)	Certification is available through the Certification Board for Music Therapists (CBMT). No formal licensure process is available. Many trained practitioners incorporate music therapy into their practice.	Certification requires the completion of an academic and clinical training program approved by the American Music Therapy Association and completion of a written examination. CBMT programs are accredited by the National Commission for Certifying Agencies.	CBMT www.cbmt.org
Naturopathy	ND (doctor of naturopathy)	Certification can be obtained through the Naturopathic Physicians Licensing Examination Board and the North American Board of Naturopathic Examiners. 15 states, the District of Columbia, Puerto Rico, and the U.S. Virgin Islands have licensing laws for naturopathic doctors.	Each of the six schools in North America is either accredited or is a candidate for accreditation by an agency of the U.S. Department of Education. Licensure requires graduation from a four-year, residential naturopathic medical school and passing a post-doctoral board examination.	American Association of Naturopathic Physicians www.naturopathic.org

(Continued on next page)

Table 2. Examples* of CAM Practices With Educational Preparation, Licensure, and Credentialing Criteria (Continued)

Practice	Acronym	Certification or Licensing Body	Educational Preparation	Related Links
Osteopathy	DO (doctor of osteopathy) C-NMM/OMM, FAAO (certified neuromusculo-skeletal medicine and osteopathic manipulative medicine, fellow in the American Academy of Osteopathy)	The American Osteopathic Association has 18 certifying bodies. The two levels of certification are general certification in neuromusculoskeletal medicine and osteopathic manipulative medicine (C-NMM/OMM) and fellowship in the American Academy of Osteopathy (FAAO).	A number of osteopathic medical schools operate in the United States. Three specialty training programs exist: (1) two-year program in NMM/OMM; (2) one-year program in NMM and OMM followed by completion of an American Osteopathic Association–approved residency in another discipline, and (3) integrated three-year program in family practice and NMM and OMM.	American Academy of Osteopathy www.academyofosteopathy.org
Reflexology	None at this time	Certification is available through the American Reflexology Certification Board (ARCB). ARCB does not accredit schools, instructors, or curricula. Many trained practitioners incorporate reflexology into their practice.	A number of reflexology programs are available in the United States. Educational programs vary with introductory programs that include less than 100 hours of study to advanced programs with more than 100 hours of study.	ARCB http://arcb.net

(Continued on next page)

Table 2. Examples* of CAM Practices With Educational Preparation, Licensure, and Credentialing Criteria *(Continued)*

Practice	Acronym	Certification or Licensing Body	Educational Preparation	Related Links
Reiki	RP (Reiki practitioner) RMT (registered massage therapist)	Certification is available through several groups, such as the American Board of Holistic Practitioners. No formal licensure process exists. Many trained practitioners incorporate Reiki into their practice.	Training in traditional Reiki has three levels: First and second levels can be given in 8–12-hour classes over two weekends. Third-level training to become a Reiki master may be completed in three days.	International Association of Reiki Professionals www.iarp.org
Yoga	None at this time	Certification is available through the Yoga Alliance. No formal licensure process exists. Many trained practitioners incorporate yoga into their practice.	Yoga schools train individuals to become yoga instructors, and with 200 hours of training, instructors can become certified.	Yoga Alliance www.yogaalliance.org

*This is not a definitive guide to CAM certification bodies, licensing laws, and education preparation of these providers. The information presented here is current at the time of printing and serves as examples only. Refer to your state licensing boards or professional associations for more information.

Table 3. Grading Strength and Quality of Recommendations for CAM Therapies

Source	Strength of Study Design	Strength of End Points Measured	Level of Evidence Score
Natural Medicines Comprehensive Database www.naturaldatabase.com	Weight of evidence ○ Low ○○ Moderate ○○○ High Direction of Evidence ⇑ Clearly positive ⇗ Tentatively positive ⇒ Uncertain ⇘ Tentatively negative ⇓ Clearly negative Serious Safety Concerns YES Serious events have been reported or are considered possible NO Reports of serious events were not located and are considered unlikely		Weight of evidence Direction of evidence Serious safety concerns
Natural Standard Database www.naturalstandard.com	A Strong scientific evidence B Good scientific evidence C Unclear or conflicting scientific evidence D Fair negative scientific evidence F Strong negative scientific evidence Lack of Evidence Unable to evaluate efficacy due to lack of adequate human data	Quality of Study 0–2 Poor 3–4 Good 5 Excellent	A B C D F Lack of Evidence
Physician Data Query www.cancer.gov/cancer topics/pdq/cam	1 Randomized clinical trials (RCT) (double-blinded and nonblinded) (DB/NB) 2 Non-RCT 3 Case series 4 Best case series	A Total Mortality B CS-Mortality C QOL D Indirect Surrogates	1–4 joined with A-D Joining score for study design with strength of end points measured

Note. From "Cancer Complementary and Alternative Medicine From the Patient, Provider, and Community Viewpoints. Part 2: Examining CAM Options in Conventional Biomedical Cancer Care," by C.O. Lee, 2004. Retrieved December 22, 2009, from http://static.capitalreach.com/o/ons/2004iol/3506/Lee.pdf. Copyright Colleen O. Lee. Adapted with permission.

Table 4. Examples of Efficacy and Safety of CAM Therapies by Modality

Therapy	Description	Evidence	Side Effects	Cautions/ Contraindications
		Alternative Medical Systems		
Homeopathy	Whole system of medicine that uses highly diluted substances to induce the body's self-healing mechanisms to bring about symptom or disease resolution (Jonas & Jacobs, 1996).	NS: Insufficient reliable evidence available for "Strong," "Good," and "Fair Negative" scientific evidence ratings; "Unclear or Conflicting Evidence" rating for menopausal symptoms/hot flashes in breast cancer survivors; "Unproven" rating for cancer, depression, and estrogen withdrawal in breast cancer NMCD: Insufficient reliable evidence available to provide an evidence rating. PDQ: No PDQ summary is available for this therapy.	NS: Limited safety research because therapies are often individualized. NMCD: Limited safety research because therapies are often individualized. There are no published reports of serious adverse effects. PDQ: N/A	NS: No published reports of serious adverse effects were found NMCD: There are no published reports of serious adverse effects. PDQ: N/A

(Continued on next page)

Table 4. Examples of Efficacy and Safety of CAM Therapies by Modality (Continued)

Therapy	Description	Evidence	Side Effects	Cautions/ Contraindications
		Alternative Medical Systems		
Naturopathy	Combines conventional medical understanding of human physiology and disease with alternative therapies aimed at stimulating the body's own ability over drugs and surgery. These therapies may include herbal and nutritional therapies, acupuncture, bodywork and body movement, hydrotherapy, meditation, and counseling.	NS: No randomized clinical studies show the effectiveness of naturopathic medicine as a whole. NMCD: No randomized clinical studies show the effectiveness of naturopathic medicine as a whole. PDQ: None available	NS: None reported NMCD: None reported PDQ: N/A	NS: None reported NMCD: None reported PDQ: N/A

(Continued on next page)

Table 4. Examples of Efficacy and Safety of CAM Therapies by Modality (Continued)

Therapy	Description	Evidence	Side Effects	Cautions/ Contraindications
		Alternative Medical Systems		
Traditional Chinese Medicine	Acupuncture is a family of procedures involving the stimulation of anatomical points (acupoints) on the skin	NS: Strong—Chronic pain, postoperative pain; Good—CINV, postoperative nausea and vomiting in adults; Unclear or conflicting—anxiety, vasomotor symptoms in breast cancer, cancer pain, chemotherapy-induced leukopenia, depression, xerostomia, erectile dysfunction, insomnia, menopausal symptoms, postoperative nausea and vomiting in children, weight loss; Fair negative—smoking cessation NMCD: Possibly effective—back pain, CINV; Insufficient reliable evidence to rate—cancer-related pain, depression, smoking cessation PDQ: RCT (double-blinded, non-blinded)—four RCTs investigating acupuncture on immune system response (leukocyte activity, levels of IL-2, natural killer cells, T-cell, soluble IL-2R, and beta-endorphins) range from 1C to 1D; three RCTs investigating acupuncture on cancer-related pain are all 1C; eight RCTs investigating acupuncture for CINV are all 1C; one RCT for other cancer treatment–related symptoms (weight loss, cough, hemoptysis, others)	NS: Pneumothorax, blood clots, ruptured artery, bleeding, abscesses, cerebrospinal fluid fistula, and diabetic ketoacidosis NMCD: Dizziness, nausea and vomiting, pain, fainting, and infection of the needle insertion points PDQ: Pain or irritation at needle sites, hematoma, fatigue, lightheadedness, drowsiness; reports of infection and hepatitis	NS: Avoid in patients with valvular heart disease, bleeding disorders, anticoagulant therapy, pregnancy, systemic or local infections, pain of unknown medical origin, skin regions that have had radiation. Electroacupuncture is contraindicated in people with arrhythmia or pacemakers. Caution in pulmonary disease, older adults or medically compromised patients, and those with a medical history of seizures or vascular compromise. NMCD: None stated PDQ: None stated

(Continued on next page)

Table 4. Examples of Efficacy and Safety of CAM Therapies by Modality (Continued)

Therapy	Description	Evidence	Side Effects	Cautions/ Contraindications
		Energy Therapies		
Qigong	A traditional Chinese therapy that can be a self-trained exercise or applied by a qigong practitioner incorporating moderate intensity exercise, movements, posture, meditation, and breathing. The several varieties of qigong include tai chi, meditation, yoga, and Reiki.	NS: Strong—none reported; Good—depression, chronic pain; Unclear or Conflicting—immune function, leukopenia, QOL, stress; Unproven—anxiety, cancer prevention, cancer treatment, improved sleep NMCD: Possibly Effective—depression, pain, stress; Insufficient Reliable Evidence to Rate—none reported PDQ: No PDQ summary is available for this therapy.	NS: None reported NMCD: None reported PDQ: N/A	NS: Should not be used by those with history of mental illness unless under the close supervision of a qualified practitioner; should not be used as a sole therapy for illnesses NMCD: None reported PDQ: N/A

(Continued on next page)

Table 4. Examples of Efficacy and Safety of CAM Therapies by Modality (Continued)

Therapy	Description	Evidence	Side Effects	Cautions/ Contraindications
		Energy Therapies		
Reiki	*Rei* means universal spirit and *ki* means life energy; Reiki therefore means *universal life energy*. Considered an energy therapy and a touch therapy. The Reiki practitioner is the conduit for the transmission or transfer of energy.	NS: None reported for Strong, Good, and Fair Negative ratings; Unclear or Conflicting evidence for cancer-related pain and fatigue, depression, and stress; Unproven for anemia, anxiety, BMT support, breast cancer, neuropathy, decreasing adverse events related to chemotherapy and radiation therapy. NMCD: Possibly Effective—none reported; Insufficient Reliable Evidence to Rate—cancer-related fatigue, cancer-related pain PDQ: There is no PDQ summary for this therapy	NS: None reported NMCD: None reported; anecdotal reports of patients experiencing tingling sensations, sleepiness, and relaxation PDQ: N/A	NS: None reported NMCD: Unknown PDQ: N/A

(Continued on next page)

Table 4. Examples of Efficacy and Safety of CAM Therapies by Modality (Continued)

Therapy	Description	Evidence	Side Effects	Cautions/ Contraindications
		Exercise Therapies		
Tai chi	System of movements and positions that address the mind to reduce stress and increase memory and for the body to improve posture and strength. The five major styles are Chen, Yang, Wu/Hao, Wu, and Sun.	NS: None reported for Strong, Good, and Fair Negative ratings; Unclear or Conflicting—chronic pain, depression, fatigue, exercise capacity, and sleep disorders NMCD: Possibly Effective—none reported; Insufficient Reliable Evidence to Rate—combination of tai chi plus qigong exercise improves balance in older adults; may lead to a decreased risk of falls PDQ: There is no PDQ summary for this therapy.	NS: Safe when used in patients with any medical condition in which the person is ambulatory and has no contraindication to mild exercise NMCD: Safely used in clinical trials without any evidence of adverse outcomes PDQ: N/A	NS: None reported NMCD: None reported PDQ: N/A

(Continued on next page)

Table 4. Examples of Efficacy and Safety of CAM Therapies by Modality (*Continued*)

Therapy	Description	Evidence	Side Effects	Cautions/ Contraindications
		Exercise Therapies		
Yoga	Ancient system of relaxation, exercise, and healing aimed to achieve fitness and a healthy lifestyle. Schools of practice include Hatha, Karma, Bhakti, and Raja. The Eight Limbs are pranayama (breathing exercises), asana (physical postures), yama (moral behavior), niyama (healthy habit), dharana (concentration), pratyahara (sense withdrawal), dhyana (contemplation), and samadhi (higher consciousness).	NS: Strong—hypertension; Good—anxiety, depression; Unclear or Conflicting—fatigue, headache, insomnia, memory, menopausal symptoms, muscle soreness, pain; none reported for Fair Negative rating NMCD: Possibly Effective—back pain, depression; Insufficient Reliable Evidence to Rate—anxiety, CINV, hypertension, insomnia, menopausal symptoms, migraine headaches, stress PDQ: There is no PDQ summary for this therapy.	NS: Safe in healthy and non-contraindicated health conditions with proper guidance by a qualified instructor NMCD: Likely safe when used appropriately; some aggressive forms of yoga exercises might not be safe; reports of serious adverse events have occurred in people using the pranayama and kapalabhati pranayama techniques PDQ: N/A	NS: Patients with spinal disc disease, fragile or atherosclerotic neck arteries, high or low blood pressure, glaucoma, retinal detachment, severe osteoporosis, cervical spondylitis, or if at risk for blood clots should avoid some inverted poses. NMCD: Kapalabhati pranayama may place excessive pressure on the abdomen in patients who have undergone abdominal surgery, as well as might increase blood pressure and have an adverse outcome in patients with uncontrolled hypertension. PDQ: N/A

(Continued on next page)

Table 4. Examples of Efficacy and Safety of CAM Therapies by Modality (Continued)

Therapy	Description	Evidence	Side Effects	Cautions/ Contraindications
		Manipulative and Body-Based Methods		
Massage (Swedish [most common], body-work, Rolfing® [Rolf Institute of Structural Integration], shiatsu)	Massage is a broad term encompassing a variety of approaches to the manipulation of soft tissue to achieve health benefits. Practitioners primarily use their hands but may also use their forearms, elbows, or even their feet. Lubricants often are added to reduce friction and discomfort. Massage is increasingly combined with other modalities in the development of integrative treatment programs for chronic or degenerative illness such as cancer.	NS: None reported for Strong or Fair Negative ratings; Good—cancer-related QOL; Unclear or Conflicting—anxiety, back pain, chronic pain, CINV, constipation, depression, diagnostic procedures, myofascial, stress, and use in children younger than 18 years old NMCD: Insufficient Reliable Evidence to Rate—shiatsu PDQ: There is no PDQ summary for this therapy	NS: Allergic response may occur when aromatic or topical essential oils are used with massage. NMCD: No significant clinical trials to evaluate safety. Little scientific information about safety and adverse outcomes for shiatsu. PDQ: N/A	NS: Use caution in patients with a history of sexual abuse or psychoses. Avoid eyes and areas of the body with fractures or weakened bones (from osteoporosis or cancer), opening or healing skin wounds, and skin infections, points of recent surgery, or history of blood clots. Avoid with patients with bleeding disorders, anticoagulant therapies or any other blood or circulation problems. In children younger than 18 years old, note decrease in plasma glucose. NMCD: Single report of a patient developing neck pain, dysphasia, and gait disturbances during shiatsu treatment. PDQ: N/A

(Continued on next page)

Table 4. Examples of Efficacy and Safety of CAM Therapies by Modality (Continued)

Therapy	Description	Evidence	Side Effects	Cautions/ Contraindications
		Manipulative and Body-Based Methods		
Reflexology (auricular reflexology, body reflexology, chakra energy reflexology, foot reflexology, foot acupressure, macroreflexology [ear-foot-hand], zone therapy, lymphatic reflexology)	Reflexology is based on the concept that areas of the feet correspond to other body parts, and stimulation of these areas on the feet can affect the associated body part. Some practitioners perform reflexology of the ears and hands.	NS: None reported for Strong, Good, and Fair Negative ratings; Unclear or Conflicting—anxiety, low back pain, pediatric constipation, depression, fatigue, headache, menopausal symptoms, relief of cancer-related symptoms, and cancer-related QOL NMCD: Possibly Effective—menopausal symptoms; Insufficient Reliable Evidence to Rate—chemotherapy (QOL), chronic obstructive pulmonary disease, migraine, multiple sclerosis, overactive bladder, premenstrual syndrome, tension headache PDQ: There is no PDQ summary for this therapy.	NS: Painful treatments may signify underlying foot disorder or improper technique. NMCD: Some patients report malaise, fatigue, nausea, or flu-like symptoms after treatment. PDQ: N/A	NS: Not recommended to be used alone because of lack of efficacy evidence. Use with caution in patients with diabetes, heart disease (pacemaker), unstable blood pressure, cancer, active infections, history of fainting or syncope, mental illness, gallbladder or kidney disease (based on information from reflexology texts, not scientific evidence) NMCD: None reported PDQ: N/A

(Continued on next page)

Table 4. Examples of Efficacy and Safety of CAM Therapies by Modality (Continued)

Therapy	Description	Evidence	Side Effects	Cautions/ Contraindications
Mind-Body Intervention				
Aromatherapy	Refers to several modalities that deliver essential oils to the body. Essential oils are mixed with a carrier oil or diluted in alcohol before being applied to the skin, sprayed in the air, or inhaled. Massage is a common means of delivering oils into the body through the skin.	NS: None reported for Strong, Good, and Fair Negative ratings; Unclear or Conflicting—anxiety, QOL in patients with cancer, constipation, depression, dysmenorrhea, lymphedema, postoperative nausea and vomiting, sleep quality NMCD: Possibly Effective—none reported; Possibly Ineffective— postoperative nausea; Insufficient Reliable Evidence to Rate—anxiety, depression, psychological well-being PDQ: Three RCTs showed no effect of lavender, chamomile, and massage on mood, QOL, pain or anxiety; two RCTs showed in anxiety and improved QOL with chamomile and massage; one RCT showed decreased anxiety and pain and improved mobility with an aromatherapy blend and massage.	NS: Likely safe when diluted in carrier oils and used via airborne administration in limited amounts; possibly safe when applied via massage, inunction, or bathwater in highly dilute concentrations; unsafe when taken internally or full-strength NMCD: Possibly safe when used short-term appropriately and by inhalation; possibly unsafe when used orally PDQ: Minimal adverse effects; contact dermatitis has been reported with prolonged skin contact	NS: Allergy may occur with the use of essential oils and may be caused by contamination or constituents of the herbs; avoid in patients with history of allergic dermatitis or who are operating heavy machinery NMCD: Bergamot oil can cause photosensitization; application of concentrated oil to a large skin surface or broken skin may cause allergic dermatitis. PDQ: Theoretical concern for women at high risk for hormonally sensitive breast cancer when using lavender and tea tree oils because of possible estrogenic and antiandrogenic effects

(Continued on next page)

Table 4. Examples of Efficacy and Safety of CAM Therapies by Modality (Continued)

Therapy	Description	Evidence	Side Effects	Cautions/ Contraindications
		Mind-Body Intervention		
Mindfulness meditation	A practice used to free the mind of cluttered thoughts and focus on a relaxed mental and physical state. Types of meditation include concentrative mindfulness and transcendental mindfulness. Mindfulness meditation allows the mind to experience extraneous stimuli, but there is no reaction to the stimuli.	NS: None reported for Strong and Fair Negative ratings; Good—QOL in patients with cancer, stress; Unclear or Conflicting—anxiety, chronic pain, depression, mood enhancement, sleep disorders NMCD: Possibly Effective—stress; Insufficient Reliable Evidence to Rate—anxiety disorder, back pain, hypertension PDQ: There is no PDQ summary for this therapy.	NS: Presumed safe in all medical conditions and all patients NMCD: Likely safe when used appropriately; meditation has been safely used in clinical trials. PDQ: N/A	NS: Possibly unsafe in patients with mood or personality disorders or at risk for seizures NMCD: There is no known reason to expect adverse outcomes. PDQ: N/A

(Continued on next page)

Table 4. Examples of Efficacy and Safety of CAM Therapies by Modality (Continued)

Therapy	Description	Evidence	Side Effects	Cautions/ Contraindications
Nutritional Therapeutics: Macrobiotics				
Macrobiotics	An approach to life rather than a diet, but diet is predominantly vegetarian, with emphasis on vegetables, fruits, legumes, seaweeds, with small amount white meat or fish once or twice per week. The three types are Zen, American, and integrative. Followers believe that food and food quality powerfully affect health, well-being, and happiness.	NS: None stated for Strong and Good ratings; Unclear or Conflicting—cognitive function; Unproven—menopausal symptoms NMCD: Not included in this database. PDQ: There is no PDQ summary for this therapy.	NS: Nutritional deficiencies including calcium, cobalamin (B_{12}), dietary fat, iron, manganese, protein, riboflavin (B_2), vitamin B_{12}, vitamin D, and zinc; risk for anemia, rickets, scurvy, and reduced bone mass NMCD: N/A PDQ: N/A	NS: None stated NMCD: N/A PDQ: N/A

(Continued on next page)

Table 4. Examples of Efficacy and Safety of CAM Therapies by Modality (Continued)

Therapy	Description	Evidence	Side Effects	Cautions/ Contraindications
		Pharmacologic and Biologic Treatments/Complex Natural Products		
Melatonin	Hormone synthesized endogenously in the pineal gland from the amino acid tryptophan. Primary role seems to be regulation of the body's circadian rhythm, endocrine secretions, and sleep patterns. Levels of melatonin in the blood are highest prior to bedtime.	NS: Strong—jet lag; Good—insomnia in older adults, sleep enhancement in healthy people, antioxidant, benzodiazepine tapering, thrombocytopenia, ultraviolet light skin damage protection; none reported for Unclear or Conflicting and Fair Negative categories NMCD: Likely Effective—circadian rhythm sleep disorders, sleep-wake cycle disturbances; Possibly Effective—benzodiazepine withdrawal, cluster headaches, delayed sleep phase syndrome, insomnia, jet lag, nicotine withdrawal, preoperative anxiety and sedation, thrombocytopenia; Likely Ineffective—depression; Insufficient Reliable Evidence to Rate—menopausal symptoms, migraine headache PDQ: There is no PDQ summary for this therapy	NS: Likely safe when use orally for up to two years at a dose of 5 mg daily; possibly safe when used in doses up to 40 mg for short periods of time NMCD: Likely safe when used orally or parenterally for up to two months; possibly safe when used orally and appropriately long term up to nine months; used with apparent safety in short-term clinical trials in children PDQ: N/A	NS: Possibly unsafe in patients who are taking anticoagulants or have increased risk of seizure NMCD: Melatonin may increase the effect of herbs that have antiplatelet/anticoagulant constituents and may increase risk of bleeding. Concomitant use with herbs with sedative properties might cause adverse effects such as daytime drowsiness, headache, and dizziness. PDQ: N/A

(Continued on next page)

Table 4. Examples of Efficacy and Safety of CAM Therapies by Modality *(Continued)*

Therapy	Description	Evidence	Side Effects	Cautions/ Contraindications
		Pharmacologic and Biologic Treatments/Complex Natural Products		
European mistletoe (*Viscum album, Iscador, Helixor, Eurixor, Isorel*)	One of the most widely studied CAM therapies for cancer. European mistletoe has been used in Europe in the treatment of cancer since the 1920s. Avoid confusing with American mistletoe and mistletoe from Australia, Korea, New Zealand, and others.	NS: None reported for Strong, Good, and Fair Negative ratings; Unclear or Conflicting—bladder cancer, breast cancer, cervical cancer, CNS cancer, colorectal cancer, head and neck cancer, liver cancer, lung cancer, lymphatic cancer, ovarian cancer, kidney cancer, melanoma, leukemia; Unproven—anxiety, constipation, diarrhea, sleep disorders NMCD: Possibly Effective—none reported; Insufficient Reliable Evidence to Rate— bladder cancer, breast cancer, colorectal cancer, gastric cancer; Possibly Ineffective—head and neck cancers, pancreatic cancer	NS: Erythema, hyperemia, skin burning sensation/delayed hypersensitivity reaction; alters serum glucose in diabetic patients. For *Iscador*, anorexia, malaise, depressive mood, fever, swelling at injection site, pain NMCD: Oral—vomiting, diarrhea, hypotension, intestinal cramps, sleepiness, coma, death; Subcutaneous—pain at injection site, local inflammatory reactions, anaphylaxis; IV aviscumine— fatigue, fever, nausea, vomiting, urinary frequency, pruritus, hypokalemia, and elevated liver enzymes	NS: Those with known allergy to mistletoe or any of its constituents. Patients with protein hypersensitivity and/or progressive infections, acute, highly febrile illness, thyroid disease, or glaucoma. NMCD: Aviscumine (a pure form of mistletoe lectin 1)—anaphylaxis in those with previous use of European mistletoe. PDQ: None reported

(Continued on next page)

Table 4. Examples of Efficacy and Safety of CAM Therapies by Modality (Continued)

Therapy	Description	Evidence	Side Effects	Cautions/ Contraindications
Pharmacologic and Biologic Treatments/Complex Natural Products				
European mistletoe (Viscum album, Iscador, Helixor, Eurixor, Isorel) (cont.)		PDQ: RCTs—Iscador (six RCTs, two nonrandomized controlled trials, two prospective randomized matched pair studies); Eurixor (five randomized RCTs, one phase I/II trial); Helixor (two RCTs, one nonrandomized controlled trial); other mistletoe products (two randomized trials, two nonrandomized controlled trials). At this time, evidence is insufficient to recommend the use of mistletoe as a cancer treatment outside well-designed clinical trials.	PDQ: Soreness and inflammation at injection site, headache, fever, and chills; reports of severe allergic reactions, anaphylaxis	

(Continued on next page)

Table 4. Examples of Efficacy and Safety of CAM Therapies by Modality (Continued)

Therapy	Description	Evidence	Side Effects	Cautions/ Contraindications
Pharmacologic and Biologic Treatments/Complex Natural Products				
Green tea	Tea from the *Camellia sinensis* plant that may be green, black, and oolong. Fresh leaves from the *Camellia sinensis* plant are steamed to produce green tea. Green tea and green tea extracts, such as its component EGCG, have been used to prevent and treat a variety of cancers. Usually brewed and drunk as a beverage; tea extracts can be taken in capsules and are sometimes used in skin products.	NS: None reported for Strong and Fair Negative ratings; Good— Polyphenon E® (Polyphenon Pharmaceuticals) is a proprietary extract of green tea approved in the United States for the external topical use for genital warts caused by HPV; Unclear or Conflicting—anxiety (L-theanine, amino acid found in green tea), cancer (general) remains under study, menopausal symptoms, human T-cell lymphocyte virus (decreases viral load); Unproven—adenocarcinoma, antioxidants, cancer treatment side effects, cognitive function, fibrosarcoma, immune enhancement, leukoplakia, lymphocytic leukemia, asbestos-related lung injury	NS: Stimulants related to caffeine-content— insomnia, hypertension, tachycardia, incontinence; increased stomach acid production, ulcer symptoms, and sodium and potassium loss related to diuretic effect. The tannin in the tea is associated with microcytic and iron-deficiency anemia. Either increases or decreases serum glucose; decreases circulating estrogen; contains vitamin K properties and can alter anticoagulants and antiplatelet agents; Polyphenon E may cause local irritation.	NS: Effects related to caffeine-related content of green tea; potential drug interactions that cause increased stimulant effect (nicotine, ephedrine, beta-agonists, theophylline levothyroxine); potential drug interactions that cause a depressant effect (benzodiazepines). Other effects include risk of lithium toxicity with abrupt cessation of caffeine; increased aspirin and phenobarbital levels (cause unclear); increased headache relieving effect of analgesic-containing products. Dexamethasone interferes with caffeine levels (lowers the caffeine level). Drugs that increase caffeine blood levels include disulfiram, oral contraceptives, hormone replacement therapy, ciprofloxacin, norfloxacin, fluvoxamine, cimetidine, verapamil

(Continued on next page)

Table 4. Examples of Efficacy and Safety of CAM Therapies by Modality (*Continued*)

Therapy	Description	Evidence	Side Effects	Cautions/ Contraindications
Pharmacologic and Biologic Treatments/Complex Natural Products				
Green tea (*cont.*)		NMCD: Possibly Safe—orally (extract for six months containing 7% caffeine), for children in amounts commonly found in foods and beverages; Possibly Unsafe—orally for long term, doses greater than 250–350 mg/day containing caffeine; Likely Unsafe—orally at very high doses (10–14 g/day); Likely Effective—green tea extract ointment for genital warts; Possibly Effective—bladder, esophageal, pancreatic, ovarian cancers. Oral or topical use may reduce cervical dysplasia caused by HPV, oral leukoplakia; Possibly Ineffective—colorectal cancer; Insufficient Reliable Evidence to Rate—breast, gastric, lung, prostate cancers PDQ: There is no PDQ summary for this therapy.	NMCD: Nausea, vomiting, abdominal bloating and pain, dyspepsia, flatulence, diarrhea; CNS stimulation including dizziness, insomnia, fatigue, agitation, tremors, restlessness, confusion; concern about green tea extracts in capsule and beverages causing hepatotoxicity between 5–120 days; allergic reactions include cough, dyspnea, loss of consciousness, and asthma, anaphylaxis in sensitive individuals PDQ: N/A	NMCD: Anticoagulant and antiplatelet substances; green tea and bitter orange together increases blood pressure and heart rate; should not be taken with caffeine-containing herbs and supplements; green tea and ephedra together increases the risk of caffeine effects; green tea decreases the activity of folic acid; green tea reduces the absorption of non-heme iron except in older adults; antidiabetic agents interfere with blood glucose control; estrogen inhibits caffeine metabolism; therefore, serum levels increase when taken with green tea. Green tea with quinolones increases the effects of caffeine. PDQ: N/A

(Continued on next page)

Table 4. Examples of Efficacy and Safety of CAM Therapies by Modality *(Continued)*

Therapy	Description	Evidence	Side Effects	Cautions/ Contraindications
		Spiritual Therapies		
Spiritual therapies	Spiritual therapies include different approaches that can use prayer to treat or prevent illness. May include distance healing and other techniques provided in a hospice setting, at home, in a medical facility, in a residential facility, and more recently, over the Internet.	NS: None reported for Strong, Good, and Fair Negative ratings; Unclear or Conflicting—cancer, cancer-related depression, cancer-related anxiety, and cancer-related QOL NMCD: Possibly Effective—none reported; Insufficient Reliable Evidence to Rate—leukemia PDQ: Research confirms both patients and family caregivers commonly rely on spirituality and religion to help them deal with serious physical illnesses, expressing a desire to have specific spiritual and religious needs and concerns acknowledged or addressed by medical staff. Additionally, spirituality has multiple expressed forms between and within cultural and religious traditions. 28 studies representing pilot studies, meta-analysis, and prospective qualitative studies and surveys on spirituality/population/cancer site–specific research are reported.	NS: None reported NMCD: None reported PDQ: None reported	NS: Should not be used as only treatment for medical or psychiatric conditions; should not delay considerations of proven therapies; should not be used in those predisposed to self-blame or shame if desired results are not obtained NMCD: None reported PDQ: None reported

BMT—bone marrow transplant; CINV—chemotherapy-induced nausea and vomiting; CNS—central nervous system; HPV—human papillomavirus; N/A—not applicable; NS—Natural Standard Database; NMCD—Natural Medicines Comprehensive Database; PDQ—Physician Data Query; QOL—quality of life; RCTs—randomized controlled trials (double-blinded, nonblinded)

Note. Based on information from Jonas & Jacobs, 1996; National Cancer Institute, n.d.; Natural Medicines Comprehensive Database, n.d.; Natural Standard Database, n.d.

References

Angel, M., & Kassirer, J.P. (1998). Alternative medicine—the risks of untested and unregulated remedies. *New England Journal of Medicine, 339*(12), 839–841.

Jonas, W.B., & Jacobs, J. (1996). *Healing with homeopathy: The complete guide.* New York: Warner Books.

Lee, C.O. (2009). Complementary and integrative therapies. In B.H. Gobel, S. Triest-Robertson, & W.H. Vogel (Eds.), *Advanced oncology nursing certification review and resource manual* (pp. 305–327). Pittsburgh, PA: Oncology Nursing Society.

National Cancer Institute. (n.d.). *Cancer Topics PDQ®.* Retrieved August 20, 2009, from http://www.cancer.gov/cancertopics/pdq

National Cancer Institute Office of Cancer Complementary and Alternative Medicine. (2009, October). *Categories of CAM therapies.* Retrieved December 21, 2009, from http://www.cancer.gov/cam/health_categories.html

National Institutes of Health National Center for Complementary and Alternative Medicine. (2007, February). *What is CAM?* Retrieved August 27, 2009, from http://nccam.nih.gov/health/whatiscam/overview.htm

Natural Medicines Comprehensive Database. (n.d.). Retrieved August 20, 2009, from http://naturaldatabase.therapeuticresearch.com

Natural Standard Database. (n.d.). Retrieved August 20, 2009, from http://www.naturalstandard.com

Oliver, S. (2003). *Certification vs. licensure: What are the differences?* Retrieved August 27, 2009, from http://www.cbmt.org/default.asp?page=Certification vs. Licensure

SECTION IV

Herbs and Herbal Extracts

The use of herbs and dietary supplements has increased steadily in the United States. Ernst (2006) defines *herbalism* as the medical use of preparations that contain exclusively plant material. In *herbology* (a synonym for herbalism), whole plants, parts of plants, or extracts are used to prevent or treat disease. Various parts of a plant are believed to work synergistically to achieve an optimal effect. The World Health Organization (2008) estimates that 80% of the world's population uses herbal medicine for some aspect of primary health care. Patients with cancer are challenged by the symptoms related to the diagnosis of cancer and the toxicities associated with conventional cancer therapy and therefore seek what they perceive to be *natural* and *less toxic* therapies. Natural does not mean safe. Eisenberg (2001, 2002, 2003) would argue that efficacy does not justify use. His mantra, "Safety trumps efficacy," provides the guidance and wisdom needed to use herbals safely throughout the cancer symptoms and treatment experience. This means that a particular herb may be effective for a particular symptom, but if it is not safe with current medications or treatments, it should not be used in this set of circumstances (see Figures 4 and 5). Thought leaders disagree with regard to the safety of some herbs

---

Figure 4. Examples of Herbs That Alter Clotting Mechanisms

- Alfalfa
- Angelica
- Anise
- Arnica
- Asafoetida
- Bog bean
- Boldo
- Capsicum
- Carrot
- Celery
- Chamomile
- Clover
- Danshen
- Ephedra
- Fenugreek
- Feverfew
- Ginger
- Ginkgo biloba
- Ginseng
- Horse chestnut
- Licorice
- Meadowsweet
- Onion
- Papain
- Passion flower
- Poplar
- Prickly ash
- Turmeric
- Wild willow

Note. Based on information from *Physician's Desk Reference for Herbal Medicines*, 2007.

45

Figure 5. Examples of Herbs With Sedative Properties

- Calamus
- Calenda
- California poppy
- Capsicum
- Celery
- Couch grass
- Siberian ginseng
- Chamomile
- Goldenseal
- Gotu kola
- Hops
- Jamaican dogwood
- Kava
- Lemon balm
- Sage
- St. John's wort
- Skullcap
- Shepherd's purse
- Stinging nettle
- Valerian
- Wild carrot
- Withania root
- Yerba mansa
- Sassafras

Note. Based on information from *Physician's Desk Reference for Herbal Medicines,* 2007.

and natural products before, during, and after cancer therapy.

Evidence indicates that use of herbal and natural products to protect against cancer is as high as 89% among all patients and consumers (Eisenberg et al., 1993, 1998; Ernst, 2000a, 2000b; Ernst & Cassileth, 1998; Montbriand, 1997, 2000; Sparber et al., 2000; Sparber & Wootton, 2001; White, 2002). Research has shown that only 3% of HCPs believed that they have adequate information or knowledge to provide patients with information about these products (Montbriand, 2004a, 2004b). Interestingly, 97% of these HCPs reported that they were willing to be a resource if they could have reliable, evidence-based information readily available. Montbriand described herbs or natural products that have the evidence-based potential to protect against cancer growth (see Table 5).

In a review article, Montbriand (2004a) offered preliminary evidence-based information concerning those herbs or natural products that have the potential to increase cancer growth or recurrence (see Table 6). One's belief systems, age, gender, socioeconomic status, educational background, advice of peers, and previous experience with illness, cancer, and herbal use will affect the choice of herbs. The cancer experience provides a motivation to venture outside one's comfort zone, especially when supported or encouraged by family and friends. Culture may influence a choice of herbs as well. Although much needs to be learned about all CAM therapies, significant gains have occurred in the knowledge base. This expansion of knowledge with regard to herbs has been notable (see Appendix IV). Reliable resources regarding herbal medicines are available to patients and HCPs and are included in Appendix V. One gain in knowledge has been in identifying the herbs most commonly used inside and outside the United States. A number of surveys describe and list the most commonly used herbs.

Lee (2005) stated that drug interactions are a continuing concern in the pharmacologic management of cancer treatment. Drug interactions are classified as pharmaceutical, pharmacodynamic, or pharmacokinetic.

Table 5. Herbs and Natural Products With the Potential to Stop Cancer Growth

Herb or Natural Product	Scientific Name
Alpha-linolenic acid	—
American pawpaw	*Asimina triloba*
Apple	*Malus sylvestris*
Asparagus	*Asparagus officinalis*
Barley	*Hordeum distichum* or *Hordeum vulgare*
Beta-sitosterol	22,23-dihydrostigmasterol 24-beta-ethyl-delta-5-cholesten-3beta-ol 24-ethyl-cholesterol 3-beta-stigmast-5-en-3-ol
Bifidobacteria	*Bifidobacterium adolescentis* *Bifidobacterium bifidum*
Black seed	*Nigella sativa*
Blond psyllium	*Plantago ovata* *Plantago decumbens* *Plantago isphagula*
Blueberry	*Vaccinium angustifolium*
Cabbage	*Brassica oleracea*
Chrysanthemum	*Anthemis grandiflorum* *Anthemis stipulacea* *Chrysanthemum morifolium* *Dendranthema morifolium* *Matricaria morifolia*
Canthaxanthin	4,4-diketo-beta-carotene Beta, beta-carotene-4,4-dione
Chaparral	*Larrea divaricata* *Larrea tridentate*
Choline	*Trimethylethanolamine* *Beta-hydroxyethyl trimethylammonium hydroxide*
Conjugated linoleic acid	—
Cranberry	*Vaccinium macrocarpon*
Folic acid	*Pterolglutamic acid*
Forskolin	17beta-acetoxy-8,13-epoxy-1alpha

(Continued on next page)

Table 5. Herbs and Natural Products With the Potential to Stop Cancer Growth *(Continued)*

Herb or Natural Product	Scientific Name
Fructo-oligosaccharides	*Beta-D-fructofuranosidase*
Garlic	*Allium sativum*
Glucomannan	*Amorphophallus konjac*
Green tea	*Camellia sinensis*
Indole-3-carbinol	*Indole-3-methanol*
Jiaogulan	*Gynostemma pentaphyllum*
Lavender	*Lavandula angustifolia*
Lutein	*Beta, epsilon-carotene-3, 31-dio*
Lycopene	*All-trans-lycopene* and *psi-psi-carotene*
MGN-3	–
Microalgae	3,3'-dihydroxy-4,4'-diketo-beta-carotene 3S, 3'S-astaxanthin 3'R-astaxanthin and 3R,3'S-astaxanthin
MSM	Methylsulfonylmethane Dimethylsulfone
Olive oil	*Olea europae*
Peanut oil	*Arachis hypogaea*
Propolis	–
Quercetin	3,3',4'5,7-pentahydroxyflavone
Rice bran	*Oryza sativa*
Shark cartilage	*Squalus acanthias*

Note. Based on information from Montbriand, 2004b.

Pharmaceutical interactions occur following an incompatibility either physically with equipment or chemically with the agent. When taxanes precipitate in diluted fluids possessing a low pH, a pharmaceutical interaction has occurred. Pharmacodynamic interactions occur following a synergistic, additive, or antagonistic reaction as may happen in multi-drug chemotherapy regimens. Pharmacokinetic interactions occur as a result of changes in the absorption, distribution, metabolism, or elimination of a drug. Frequently, metabolizing enzymes are involved in this pro-

Table 6. Herbs or Natural Products With the Potential to Increase Cancer Growth or Recurrence

Herb or Natural Product	Scientific Name
Aletris	*Aletris farinose*
Alfalfa	*Medicago sativa*
Androstenedione	4-androstene-3, 17-dione
Anise	*Pimpinella anisum*
Black tea	*Camillia sinensis*
Boron	–
Chasteberry	*Vitex agnus-castus*
Coenzyme Q-10	*Ubiquinone, ubidecarenone, and mitoquinone*
Cohosh: Black cohosh Blue cohosh	*Cimicifuga racemosa* *Caulophyllum thalictroides*
Deer velvet	*Cervus nippon* *Cervus elaphus*
DHEA	*Dehydroepiandrosterone*
Dong quai	*Angelica sinensis*
Fennel	*Foeniculum vulgare*
Flaxseed	*Linum usitatissimum*
Ginseng: American ginseng Panax ginseng Siberian ginseng	*Panax quinquefolius* *Panax ginseng* *Eleutheroccus senticosus* or *Acanthopanax senticosus*
Glucosamine: Glucosamine hydrochloride Glucosamine sulfate N-acetyl glucosamine	2-amino-2-deoxyglucose hydrochloride 2-amino-2-deoxyglucose sulfate 2-acetamido-2-deoxyglucose
Hydrazine sulfate	–
Kefir	–

(Continued on next page)

Herb or Natural Product	Scientific Name
Lactobacillus	*Lactobacillus acidophilus* *Lactobacillus brevis* *Lactobacillus bulgaricus* *Lactobacillus casei sp. Rhamnosus* *Lactobacillus delbrueckii* *Lactobacillus fermentum* *Lactobacillus plantarum* *Lactobacillus rhamnosus*
Licorice	*Glycyrrhiza glabra*
Milk thistle	*Silybum marianum* or *Carduus marianum*
Pregnenolone	(3beta)-3-hydroxypregn-5-en-20-one
Progesterone	4-pregnene-3
Raspberry leaf	*Rubus idaeus*
Red clover	*Trifolium pretense*
Scarlet pimpernel	*Anagallis arvensis*
Star anise	*Illicium verum*
Vitamin C (high dose)	Ascorbic acid
Wild yam	*Discorea villosa*

Table 6. Herbs or Natural Products With the Potential to Increase Cancer Growth or Recurrence *(Continued)*

Note. Based on information from Montbriand, 2004a.

cess. The cytochrome P450 hepatic enzyme system is the predominant site for most drug metabolism and the site for most drug-drug interactions, including herb–cytotoxic drug interactions. More than 100 isoenzymes (also known as substrates) of cytochrome P450 exist. Enzymes responsible for the majority of drug metabolism are CYP3A (50%), CYP2D (25%), and CYP2C (20%). Cytotoxic agents are metabolized mainly involving the CYP3A isoenzyme. Some herbs are metabolized through this same pathway. The impact of herb–cytotoxic agent interactions may be an underdosing or overdosing of the anticancer agent or inducing resistance to the agent and affecting its therapeutic effect (Sparreboom, Cox, Acharya, & Figg, 2004). Oncology nurses and other HCPs play a critical role in identifying and averting potential interactions, and this is accomplished through a comprehensive medication assessment including prescription and nonprescription medications in oral (liquid or solid), topical, vaginal, rectal, eye or ear, and inhalation forms.

Oncology nurses want to be able to access and provide reliable information so that they may assist their patients in making an informed decision about the use of any CAM therapy. Herbal products are of magnified importance because they have the potential to interact with drugs being used to treat the cancer, cancer treatment side effects, and comorbidities. The American Herbal Products Association rating system classifies herbal products according to their relative safety and potential toxicity based on four categories (see Table 7).

Even with the large gains in knowledge, drug-to-herb or drug-to-supplement interactions continue to be a focus of pharmacologic management of many diseases and conditions, including cancer. When patients take herbs concurrently with cytotoxic agents, pharmacodynamics are possible that exceed our current understanding. See Table 8 for a snapshot view of some commonly used herbs, purported uses, potential side effects including the impact on laboratory tests, precautions and contraindications, and safety category. Table 9 provides known drug-supplement interactions, and Figure 6 lists herbs that may interfere with diagnostics and treatment.

Table 7. Herbal Products Rating System	
Rating	**Description**
Class 1	Herbs that can be consumed safely when used appropriately
Class 2	Herbs for which the following restrictions apply, unless otherwise directed by a qualified expert
2a	For external use only
2b	Not to be used during pregnancy
2c	Not to be used while nursing
2d	Other
Class 3	Herbs for which significant data exist to recommend this labeling, "To be used only under the supervision of an expert qualified in the appropriate use of this substance." Labeling must include proper use information as follows: dosage, contraindications, potential adverse effects and drug interactions, and any other relevant information related to the safe use of the substance.
Class 4	Herbs for which insufficient data are available for classification.

Note. From *American Herbal Products Association's Botanical Safety Handbook* (p. v), by M. McGuffin, C. Hobbs, R. Upton, and A. Goldberg (Eds.), 1997, Boca Raton, FL: CRC Press. Copyright 1997 by CRC Press. Reprinted with permission.

Table 8. Commonly Used Herbs

Herb	Purported Properties/Actions	Availability	Potential Side Effects	Precautions/Contraindications	Category*
Aloe *Aloe vera*	• Antiseptic • Laxative • Anti-inflammatory • Antiviral • Wound healing	Capsules, extract, powder, cream, gel, shampoo, conditioner	• May increase risk of hypogly-cemia if given concurrently with diabetic agents • Risk of hypokalemia if taken concurrently with licorice • May alter serum potassium (laxative properties) • May decrease serum glucose	• Inflammatory bowel disease, fecal impaction, appendicitis, abdominal pain of unknown origin • Any spasmodic gastrointestinal complaint, arrhythmia, neuropathy, edema • Bone deterioration with long-term use • Concurrent use with digoxin can cause digoxin toxicity	2b
Bilberry *Vaccinium myrtillus*	• Astringent • Tonic • Antioxidant and antiseptic • Wound healing • Antiulcer • Vasoprotective	Capsules, fluid extract, fresh berries, dried berries, liquid, tincture, dried root, dried leaves	• May cause bleeding, heart-burn, hypoglycemia, hyper-tension • May decrease serum glucose	• Increased risk of bleeding in individuals who are taking anticoagulants, anti-platelets, thrombolytic agents, or low-molecular-weight heparins	4
Chamomile *Matricaria recutita*	• Anxiolytic • Mild hypnotic • Hypoglycemic effect • Estrogen-dependent and estrogen-independent effects	Capsules, cream, fluid extract, lotion, shampoo, conditioner, tea, tincture, cosmetics	• Topical use: burning of the face, eyes, and mucous membranes • Systemic use: hypersensitivity and contact dermatitis, bruising, confusion, drowsiness, anaphylaxis	• Increased risk of bleeding with concurrent use with aspirin, antiplatelet agents, heparin, nonsteroidal anti-inflammatory drugs, warfarin, thrombin inhibitors, thrombolytics, darunavir • Caution when used concurrently with acetaminophen combination products	1

(Continued on next page)

Table 8. Commonly Used Herbs *(Continued)*

Herb	Purported Properties/Actions	Availability	Potential Side Effects	Precautions/Contraindications	Category*
Chamomile *Matricaria recutita* (cont.)	• Antispasmodic • Antimicrobial			• Increased risk of sedation with benzodiazepines, dextromethorphan/pseudoephedrine combination products, cannabinoids, ethanol, gotu kola, kava, muscle relaxants, all selective serotonin reuptake inhibitors, all sedatives and hypnotics • Increased risk of bleeding and sedation with concurrent use with capsaicin, dong quai, primrose oil, fenugreek, feverfew, fish oil, garlic, ginger, ginkgo, ginseng, horse chestnut, licorice, St. John's wort	
Cinnamon *Cinnamomum cassia*	• Antifungal • Analgesic • Antiseptic • Antidiarrheal • Antiviral • Antidiabetic (insulin potentiator) Also used for • Hypertension • Loss of appetite • Bronchitis	Dried bark, essential oil, leaves, fluid extract, powder, tincture	• Flushing, tachycardia, stomatitis, glossitis, gingivitis • Increased gastrointestinal mobility, anorexia • Allergic dermatitis • Shortness of breath • Hypersensitivity	• Avoid prolonged use in those with intestinal or gastric ulcers	2b

(Continued on next page)

Table 8. Commonly Used Herbs (Continued)

Herb	Purported Properties/Actions	Availability	Potential Side Effects	Precautions/Contraindications	Category*
Dong quai (Chinese Angelica) *Angelica sinensis*	• Menstrual irregularities and menopausal symptoms • Headache • Neuralgia • Herpes infections • Malaria	Capsules, fluid extract, powder, tablets, tea, tincture Primarily a combination product	• Nausea, vomiting, diarrhea, anorexia • Increased menstrual flow • Hypersensitivity reactions • Photosensitivity • Fever, sweating • Bleeding • May alter activated partial thromboplastin time (APTT), prothrombin time (PT), and international normalized ratio (INR)	• Increased effect of anticoagulants, antiplatelets, estrogens, and hormonal contraceptives • Increased risk of bleeding when taken concurrently with chamomile, dandelion, horse chestnut, red clover, St. John's wort • Photosensitivity when taken concurrently with St. John's Wort • Altered PT and INR • Increased central nervous system (CNS) depression and muscle relaxation with concurrent use with benzodiazepines • Hypoglycemia with concurrent use with tolbutamide	2b
Garlic *Allium sativum*	• Antimicrobial • Antilipidemic • Antitriglyceride • Antiplatelet • Antioxidant	Capsules, extract, fresh garlic, oil, powder, syrup, tablets, tea	• Halitosis • Altered coagulation • Altered serum glucose • Kyolic® (Wakunaga of America Co., Ltd.) garlic has less impact on serum glucose • Enteric-coated product lessens halitosis • May decrease low-density lipoprotein, triglycerides, and serum lipid profile • May increase PT, INR, and serum IgE	• Avoid with dacarbazine (CYP 2E 1 inhibition) • Preop/postop (alters coagulation) • Caution with other chemotherapy (data are inconclusive)	2b

(Continued on next page)

Table 8. Commonly Used Herbs (Continued)

Herb	Purported Properties/Actions	Availability	Potential Side Effects	Precautions/Contraindications	Category*
Ginkgo *Ginkgo biloba*	• Cognitive enhancement • Peripheral vascular insufficiency • Antioxidant • Enhances circulation throughout the body • Antiarthritic and analgesic	Capsules, fluid extract, tablets, tinctures	• Allergic reactions • Altered coagulation • Anxiety/restlessness • Bleeding • Gastrointestinal disturbances • Insomnia • Skin reactions • Transient headache • May increase C-peptide concentrations and plasma insulin levels	• Caution with camptothecin, cyclophosphamide, epidermal growth factor receptor—tyrosine kinase (EGFR-TK) inhibitors, epipodophyllotoxins, taxanes, vinca alkaloids (CYP3A4 and CYP2C19 inhibition) • Discourage with alkylating agents, antitumor antibiotics, and platinum analogs (free radical scavenging) • Subarachnoid hemorrhage without trauma has been associated with ginkgo • One case reported of acute CNS depression in a woman taking trazodone	1
Grape seed extract	• Antioxidant • Enhances circulation throughout the body • Decreases visual stress	Capsules, tablets, drops, liquid concentrate, cream	• Dizziness • Nausea, anorexia • Rash • Theoretically: hepatotoxicity	• Potential interactions with anticoagulant and antiplatelets (increases risk of bleeding) • Caution with camptothecin, cyclophosphamide, EGFR-TK inhibitors, epipodophyllotoxins, vinca alkaloids (CYP3A4 inhibition) • Discourage with alkylating agents, antitumor antibiotics, and platinum analogs (free radical scavenging)	4

(Continued on next page)

Table 8. Commonly Used Herbs *(Continued)*

Herb	Purported Properties/Actions	Availability	Potential Side Effects	Precautions/Contraindications	Category*
Kava *Piper meth-ysticum*	• Anti-inflammatory	Capsules, beverage, extract, tab-lets, tincture	• Hyper-reflexivity • Drowsiness • Blurred vision • Nausea, vomiting, anorexia, weight loss • Potential decrease in plate-lets, lymphocytes, bilirubin, protein, and albumin • Increase in red blood cell vol-ume • Hypersensitivity reactions • Shortness of breath (pulmo-nary hypertension) • Potential hepatotoxicity • May increase hepatic function tests: aspartate aminotrans-ferase (AST), alanine amin-otransferase (ALT), and lac-tate dehydrogenase • Chronic use associated with decreased lymphocyte count, decreased platelet size, and hematuria • May decrease albumin, biliru-bin, and total protein	• Avoid with antiparkinsonian drugs (in-creases the symptoms of Parkinson disease) • Avoid with antipsychotic medications (may cause neuroleptic movement dis-orders) • Avoid with barbiturates (increases se-dation) • Avoid with benzodiazepines (increases risk of sedation and/or coma) • Avoid with CNS depressants (increas-es sedation) • Avoid with CYP1A2, CYP2C9, CYP2C19, CYP2D6, CYP3A4 sub-strates (significantly decreases these substrates) • Oncology-specific guidelines: Avoid in all patients with existing liver disease, evidence of hepatic damage, herb-induced hepatotoxicity, in combination with hepatotoxic chemotherapy	2b; 2c; 2d

(Continued on next page)

Table 8. Commonly Used Herbs (Continued)

Herb	Purported Properties/Actions	Availability	Potential Side Effects	Precautions/Contraindications	Category*
Milk thistle *Silybum marianum*	• Hallucinogenic • Hepatoprotective • Cirrhosis of the liver caused by alcohol or virus • Anti-inflammatory • Antioxidant • Nephroprotective	Tincture, capsules	• Headache • Nausea, vomiting, diarrhea, anorexia, abdominal bloating, abdominal pain • Menstrual changes • Hypersensitivity reactions • Erectile dysfunction • Pruritus • Joint pain • May decrease AST, ALT, alkaline phosphatase, and serum glucose	• Avoid with warfarin • Avoid with combination products involving acetaminophen, dextromethorphan, pseudoephedrine, estrogen/progestin • May decrease levels of irinotecan, lorazepam, lovastatin, morphine, meprobamate	1
Purple coneflower *Echinacea purpurea*	• Antiviral • Immunostimulants • Vulvovaginal candidiasis • Psoriasis • Allergic rhinitis	Capsule, fluid extract, juice, dried powdered extract, sublingual tablets, tea, tincture	• Hepatotoxicity • Acute asthma attack • Anaphylaxis, angioedema • May increase ALT, AST, lymphocyte counts, serum IgE, erythrocyte sedimentation rate (ESR)	• Do not use in children younger than 2 years old • Avoid use in cytochrome P450 3A4 substrates such as immune-modulators (cyclosporine, protease inhibitors, corticosteroids, methotrexate) • Altered ALT, AST, lymphocytes, IgG, and ESR	1

(Continued on next page)

Table 8. Commonly Used Herbs *(Continued)*

Herb	Purported Properties/Actions	Availability	Potential Side Effects	Precautions/Contraindications	Category*
Valerian *Valeriana officinalis*	• Antianxiety • Anti-insomnia	Capsules, brewed herb, extract, tablets, tea, tincture, in combination products with other herbs	• Insomnia • Headaches • Restlessness • Nausea, vomiting, anorexia • Hepatotoxicity • Hypersensitivity reactions • Vision changes • Palpitations • May increase ALT, AST, gamma-glutamyl transferase, total bilirubin, alkaline phosphatase, and urine bilirubin	• Increased CNS depression (alcohol, barbiturates, benzodiazepines, opiates, sedatives/hypnotics) • Negates therapeutic effects of monoamine oxidase, phenytoin, warfarin • Avoid in patients with preexisting liver disease • Caution with tamoxifen (CYP2C9 inhibition) • Caution with cyclophosphamide, teniposide (CYP2C19)	1

* Classification is for the general population; not cancer-specific.

Note. Based on information from McGuffin et al., 1997; Natural Standard Database, n.d.; *Physician's Desk Reference for Herbal Medicines*, 2007; Skidmore-Roth, 2010.

Table 9. Potential Drug-Herb-Vitamin-Mineral Interactions

Herb/Vitamin/Mineral	Interaction
Alcohol (Ethanol)	
Beta-carotene	Decreased by alcohol
Black cohosh	Increased risk of hepatotoxicity
Capsicum annuum (oral capsaicin)	Increased risk of sedation
Chamomile (German)	Increased risk of sedation
Goldenseal	May increase the sedative effects of alcohol
Gotu kola	Increased risk of sedation
Hawthorn	Increased central nervous system (CNS) depression
Hops	Increased CNS depression
Kava	Increased risk of hepatotoxicity, sedation, psychomotor impairment
Lemon balm	Increased risk of sedation
Melatonin	Increased risk of sedation
St. John's wort	May increase monoamine oxidase inhibition; avoid concurrent use
Lavender	Increased sedation when used with aromatherapy and drugs or herbs that cause sedation; avoid concurrent use
Valerian	Increased risk of sedation
Willow bark	Increased risk of gastrointestinal bleeding (willow bark contains salicylates)
Angiotensin-Converting Enzyme Inhibitors	
Black cohosh	Increased risk of hepatotoxicity
Capsaicin (topical)	Increased risk of clot formation
Kava	Increased risk of hepatotoxicity
St. John's wort	May lead to severe photosensitivity; avoid concurrent use
Yohimbe	May decrease or block actions of these drugs; avoid concurrent use

(Continued on next page)

Table 9. Potential Drug-Herb-Vitamin-Mineral Interactions *(Continued)*

Herb/Vitamin/Mineral	Interaction
Antacids, Histamine 1 (H_1)/ Histamine 2 (H_2) Blockers, Proton Pump Inhibitors (PPIs)	
Acidophilus	Antacids should be taken 30–60 minutes before acidophilus.
Angelica	May increase stomach acid, which may decrease the antacid action and may decrease PPI action
Beta-carotene	May decrease the action of PPIs
Capsicum	May decrease efficacy of H_2 blockers; may decrease the action of PPIs
Cascara	Antacids may decrease the action of cascara if taken within one hour of the herb.
Chromium picolinate	May decrease serum chromium levels
Dandelion	May decrease the action of antacids, H_2 blockers, and PPIs
Devil's claw	May decrease the action of antacids, H_2 blockers, and PPIs
Ginger	May decrease efficacy of H_2 blockers; may decrease the action of PPIs
Goldenseal	May decrease efficacy of H_2 blockers; may decrease the action of PPIs
Lavender	Risk for sedation; avoid concurrent use with H_1 blockers
Peppermint	PPIs and antacids may cause premature dissolution of enteric-coated peppermint oil capsules.
Antibiotics	
Acidophilus and antibiotics (general)	Avoid concurrent use; space by at least two hours
Fennel and ciprofloxacin	Affects the absorption, distribution, and elimination of ciprofloxacin; dosages should be spaced by at least two hours
St. John's wort and levofloxacin and trimethoprim-sulfamethoxazole	May increase risk of skin photosensitivity
Ephedra and levofloxacin	May increase risk of cardiac arrhythmia (QT prolongation)
Black cohosh and kava and trimethoprim-sulfamethoxazole	May increase risk of hepatotoxicity

(Continued on next page)

Table 9. Potential Drug-Herb-Vitamin-Mineral Interactions *(Continued)*

Herb/Vitamin/Mineral	Interaction
Anticoagulants (ACs), Warfarin, and Antiplatelet Agents (APAs)	
Acidophilus and warfarin	Decreases warfarin action
Alfalfa and warfarin	May increase prothrombin time and prolong bleeding
Allspice and APAs	May inhibit platelets, causing bleeding
Angelica and APAs	Many species increase prothrombin time and prolong bleeding; avoid concurrent use
Angelica and ACs	May prolong bleeding; avoid concurrent use
Angelica and warfarin	May increase prothrombin time and prolong bleeding
Arginine and APAs	May cause gastric irritation
Bilberry and ACs	May increase the action of ACs
Bilberry and APAs	May cause antiaggregation of platelets
Chamomile and ACs	May interfere with the actions of ACs; avoid concurrent use
Chondroitin and ACs	Can cause increased bleeding; avoid high doses of chondroitin
Cloves and ACs	May increase the effect of ACs
Cloves and APAs	May increase the effect of APAs
Coenzyme Q10 and ACs	May decrease the action of ACs; avoid concurrent use
Cranberry and warfarin	May increase international normalized ratio (INR) and increase risk of bleeding
Dandelion and APAs	May increase bleeding
Devil's claw and warfarin	May cause risk of bleeding
Feverfew and APAs	May increase the action of APAs; avoid concurrent use
Fish oil and ACs	May increase risk of bleeding; avoid concurrent use
Flax and ACs	May increase risk of bleeding; avoid concurrent use
Flax and APAs	May increase risk of bleeding
Garlic and ACs	May increase bleeding; avoid concurrent use

(Continued on next page)

Table 9. Potential Drug-Herb-Vitamin-Mineral Interactions *(Continued)*	
Herb/Vitamin/Mineral	**Interaction**
Anticoagulants (ACs), Warfarin, and Antiplatelet Agents (APAs) (cont.)	
Garlic and APAs	May increase bleeding; avoid concurrent use
Ginkgo and ACs	May increase risk of bleeding; avoid concurrent use
Ginkgo and APAs	May increase risk of bleeding; avoid concurrent use
Ginseng and ACs	May decrease the action of ACs
Ginseng and APAs	May decrease the action of APAs
Glucosamine and ACs	High levels of glucosamine can lead to bleeding risk
Glucosamine and APAs	High levels of glucosamine can lead to bleeding risk
Goldenseal and ACs	May decrease the effects of ACs
Saw palmetto and ACs	May potentiate the anticoagulant effect of salicylates; avoid concurrent use
Saw palmetto and APAs	May lead to increased bleeding; avoid concurrent use
Turmeric and APAs	May result in increased risk of bleeding; avoid concurrent use
Antidepressants and Selective Serotonin Reuptake Inhibitors (SSRIs)	
St. John's wort, Kava, valerian, and antidepressants (general)	May cause serotonin syndrome and increased risk of sedation
Bitter orange and SSRIs	Can inhibit cytochrome P450 3A4 and increase drug levels
Fenugreek and SSRIs	Increased risk of bleeding
Ginkgo and SSRIs	Often used to reverse side effects of SSRIs
St. John's wort and SSRIs	Serotonin syndrome and an additive effect may occur; may lead to coma; avoid concurrent use
Yohimbe and SSRIs	May cause increased CNS stimulation; avoid concurrent use

(Continued on next page)

Table 9. Potential Drug-Herb-Vitamin-Mineral Interactions *(Continued)*

Herb/Vitamin/Mineral	Interaction
Antidiabetic Agents	
Aloe	Internal use may increase the effects of antidiabetics.
Basil	May increase hypoglycemic effects; avoid concurrent use
Bee pollen	May decrease effectiveness of antidiabetics and increase hyperglycemia; avoid concurrent use
Bilberry	May increase hypoglycemia
Coenzyme Q10	May increase the action of coenzyme Q10 and deplete endogenous stores; avoid concurrent use
Dandelion	May increase the effects of antidiabetics; avoid concurrent use
Devil's claw	May cause an additive effect
Ephedra	May increase blood glucose
Flax	May increase the action of antidiabetics
Garlic	Because of the hypoglycemic effects of garlic, oral antidiabetic dosages may need to be adjusted.
Ginseng	May increase the hypoglycemic effects of oral antidiabetics; avoid concurrent use
Marshmallow	May increase the hypoglycemic action of antidiabetics
Sage	May increase the action of antidiabetics
Siberian ginseng	May increase levels of antidiabetics; avoid concurrent use
Antihypertensives	
Arnica	Internal use may decrease the effect of antihypertensives.
Bayberry	Bayberry's tannin may increase sodium and water retention.
Black cohosh	Increases the action of antihypertensives
Cat's claw	May increase the hypotensive effects of antihypertensives; avoid concurrent use
Celery	May increase the effects of antihypertensives
Dandelion	May increase the effects of antihypertensives; avoid concurrent use
Goldenseal	May increase the effects of antihypertensives

(Continued on next page)

Table 9. Potential Drug-Herb-Vitamin-Mineral Interactions *(Continued)*

Herb/Vitamin/Mineral	Interaction
Antihypertensives (cont.)	
Hawthorn	May increase hypotension; avoid concurrent use
Licorice	May cause increased hypokalemia; avoid concurrent use
Mistletoe, European	May increase the hypotensive effects of antihypertensives; avoid concurrent use
Yohimbe	May decrease or block the actions of these drugs; avoid concurrent use
Antineoplastics, Oral and Parenteral Chemotherapeutic Agents, and Immunosuppressants	
Acidophilus and antineoplastics	Avoid concurrent use
Acidophilus and immunosuppressants	Avoid concurrent use
Astragalus and antineoplastics	May decrease the effect of cyclophosphamide
Astragalus and immunosuppressants	May interfere with immunosuppressants
Bitter orange and immunosuppressants	Can inhibit cytochrome P450 3A4 and increase drug levels
Black cohosh and antineoplastics	May increase toxicity of doxorubicin; avoid concurrent use
Black cohosh and tamoxifen	May augment the antiproliferative properties of tamoxifen
Dehydroepiandrosterone (DHEA) and tamoxifen	Do not take together; DHEA is a potent estrogen agonist
Ginseng and immunosuppressants	May diminish the effect of immunosuppressants; do not use before, during, or after transplant surgery
Melatonin and immunosuppressants	May decrease response to immunosuppressants
Milk thistle and antineoplastics	May prevent nephrotoxicity from platinum antineoplastics
Saw palmetto and immunosuppressants	May increase or decrease immunostimulants effects; avoid concurrent use

(Continued on next page)

Table 9. Potential Drug-Herb-Vitamin-Mineral Interactions *(Continued)*

Herb/Vitamin/Mineral	Interaction
Antineoplastics, Oral and Parenteral Chemotherapeutic Agents, and Immunosuppressants	
Soy and tamoxifen	May interfere with tamoxifen absorption; avoid concurrent use
St. John's wort	May increase the antiretroviral action when taken orally in combination with indinavir
Yew and antineoplastics	May cause increased myelosuppression; avoid concurrent use
Benzodiazepines	
Bitter orange	Can inhibit cytochrome P450 3A4 and increase drug levels
Coffee	May decrease the effect of benzodiazepines
Goldenseal	May slow the metabolism of benzodiazepines
Kava	Increased sedation and coma; avoid concurrent use
Melatonin	May increase the anxiolytic effects of benzodiazepines; use cautiously
Corticosteroids	
Black cohosh	May increase effects; avoid concurrent use
Buckthorn	Hypokalemia can result from use of buckthorn with corticosteroids; avoid concurrent use.
DHEA	Corticosteroids may decrease DHEA levels.
Estrogens	
Alfalfa	May interfere with hormonal replacement therapy of contraceptives
Soy	May interfere with estrogen absorption; avoid concurrent use
Iron	
Anise	May increase the action of iron; avoid concurrent use
Bilberry	Interferes with iron absorption; avoid concurrent use

(Continued on next page)

Table 9. Potential Drug-Herb-Vitamin-Mineral Interactions *(Continued)*

Herb/Vitamin/Mineral	Interaction
Magnesium	
Melatonin	Increased inhibition of N-methyl-D-aspartate receptors; avoid concurrent use
Raspberry	Raspberry tea may decrease absorption of magnesium.
Nonsteroidal Anti-Inflammatory Drugs (NSAIDs) and Salicylates	
Bilberry and NSAIDs	May increase the action of NSAIDs
Chondroitin and NSAIDs	Can cause increased bleeding; avoid high doses of chondroitin
Dandelion and NSAIDs	May increase bleeding when used with NSAIDs
Garlic and NSAIDs	May increase bleeding; avoid concurrent use
Saw palmetto and NSAIDs	May lead to increased bleeding time; avoid concurrent use
St. John's wort and NSAIDs	May lead to severe photosensitivity; avoid concurrent use
Chondroitin and salicylates	Can cause increased bleeding; avoid high doses of chondroitin
Cloves and salicylates	May increase the effects of salicylates
Dandelion and salicylates	May increase bleeding when used with salicylates
Garlic and salicylates	May increase bleeding when used with salicylates
Ginkgo and salicylates	May increase bleeding when used with salicylates
Ginseng and salicylates	May decrease the action of salicylates

Note. Based on information from Kliewer, 2004; McGuffin et al., 1997; Natural Standard Database, n.d.; *Physician's Desk Reference for Herbal Medicines*, 2007; Skidmore-Roth, 2010.

Figure 6. Herbs That Theoretically May Interfere With Nuclear Medicine and Diagnostics

Nuclear Medicine
- Glomerular filtration rate test—fish oils, juniper, L-arginine, parsley, high-dose vitamin C
- miBG (metaiodobenzylguanidine) therapy—lobelia, ephedra, ginseng
- Somatostatin analog therapy—ginseng, ginkgo biloba
- Thyroid therapy—iodine, lithium, selenium, garlic

Diagnostics
- Black cohosh
- Wild yam
- Soy
- Valerian
- Kava
- Green tea
- Feverfew
- Milk thistle
- Anise
- Chromium
- St. John's wort

Note. Based on information from Kliewer, 2004; Natural Standard Database, n.d.; Skidmore-Roth, 2010.

References

Eisenberg, D. (2001, February). *Complementary and integrative medicine: Clinical update and implications for practice.* Boston, MA.

Eisenberg, D. (2002, March). *Complementary and integrative medicine: State of the science and clinical applications.* Boston, MA.

Eisenberg, D. (2003, March). *Ninth annual CME conference: Integrating complementary therapies into clinical practice: Cases and evidence.* Boston, MA.

Eisenberg, D.M., Davis, R.B., Ettner, S.L., Appel, S., Wilkey, S., Van Rompay, M., et al. (1998). Trends in alternative medicine in the United States, 1990–1997: Results of a follow-up national survey. *JAMA, 280*(18), 1569–1575.

Eisenberg, D.M., Kessler, R.C., Foster, C., Norlock, F.E., Calkins, D.R., & Delbanco, T.L. (1993). Unconventional medicine in the United States: Prevalence, cost, and patterns of use. *New England Journal of Medicine, 328*(4), 246–252.

Ernst, E. (2000a). Prevalence of use of complementary/alternative medicine: A systematic review. *Bulletin of the World Health Organization, 78*(2), 252–257.

Ernst, E. (2000b). The role of complementary and alternative medicine in cancer. *Lancet Oncology, 1*(3), 176–180.

Ernst, E. (2006). Herbalism. In E. Ernst, M.H. Pittler, & B. Wider (Eds.), *The desktop guide to complementary and alternative medicine* (2nd ed., pp. 319–325). Philadelphia: Elsevier Mosby.

Ernst, E., & Cassileth, B.R. (1998). The prevalence of complementary/alternative medicine in cancer: A systematic review. *Cancer, 83*(4), 777–782.

Kliewer, S.A. (2004, October). *NIH VideoCasting: Reverse herbology: Predicting and preventing adverse herb-drug interactions.* Lecture presented at the National Institute on Drug Abuse, Baltimore, MD.

Lee, C.O. (2005). Herbs and cytotoxic drugs: Recognizing and communicating potentially relevant interactions. *Clinical Journal of Oncology Nursing, 9*(4), 481–487.

McGuffin, M., Hobbs, C., Upton, R., & Goldberg, A. (1997). Herb listing by classification. In M. McGuffin, C. Hobbs, R. Upton, & A. Goldberg (Eds.), *American Herbal Products Association's botanical safety handbook* (pp. 181–190). Boca Raton, FL: CRC Press.

Montbriand, M.J. (1997). Empowerment of seniors through improved communication about medication. In L.F. Heumann (Ed.), *Proceedings of the Sixth International Conference on Systems Science in Health-Social Services for the Elderly and the Disabled* (pp. 258–264). Chicago: University of Illinois at Urbana-Champaign.

Montbriand, M.J. (2000). Alternative therapies: Health professionals' attitudes. *Canadian Nurse, 96*(3), 22–26.

Montbriand, M.J. (2004a). Herbs or natural products that increase cancer growth or recurrence: Part two of a four-part series [Online exclusive]. *Oncology Nursing Forum, 31*(5), E99–E115. Retrieved August 20, 2009, from http://ons.metapress.com/content/5281847v81675n21/fulltext.pdf

Montbriand, M.J. (2004b). Herbs or natural products that protect against cancer growth: Part three of a four-part series [Online exclusive]. *Oncology Nursing Forum, 31*(6), E127–E146. Retrieved August 20, 2009, from http://ons.metapress.com/content/d35x738211q56657/fulltext.pdf

Natural Standard Database. (n.d.). Retrieved August 20, 2009, from http://www.naturalstandard.com

Physician's Desk Reference for herbal medicines (4th ed.). (2007). Montvale, NJ: Thomson Healthcare.

Skidmore-Roth, L. (2010). *Mosby's handbook of herbs and natural supplements* (4th ed.). St. Louis, MO: Elsevier Mosby.

Sparber, A., Bauer, L., Curt, G., Eisenberg, D., Levin, T., Parks, S., et al. (2000). Use of complementary medicine by adult patients participating in cancer clinical trials. *Oncology Nursing Forum, 27*(4), 623–630.

Sparber, A., & Wootton, J.C. (2001). Surveys of complementary and alternative medicine: Part II. Use of alternative and complementary cancer therapies. *Journal of Alternative and Complementary Medicine, 7*(3), 281–287.

Sparreboom, A., Cox, M.C., Acharya, M.R., & Figg, W.D. (2004). Herbal remedies in the United States: Potential adverse interactions with anticancer agents. *Journal of Clinical Oncology, 22*(12), 2489–2503.

White, J.D. (2002). Complementary and alternative medicine research: A National Cancer Institute perspective. *Seminars in Oncology, 29*(6), 546–551.

World Health Organization. (2008, December). *Traditional medicine* [Fact Sheet No. 134]. Retrieved August 18, 2009, from http://www.who.int/mediacentre/factsheets/fs134/en

Symptom Management: Evidence of Efficacy and Safety of Commonly Used CAM Therapies by Symptom

Introduction

Symptom management spans the prediagnosis to survivorship spectrum. Tremendous advances have been made in offering relief from symptoms associated with the cancer disease process, its treatment, and the many and varied physical, emotional, spiritual, and psychological long-term consequences. Oncology nurses identify, assess, deliver symptom management interventions, and monitor long-term outcomes; pivotal publications assist nurses in providing this high level of care (Eaton & Tipton, 2009; Yarbro, Frogge, & Goodman, 2005). Additionally, Paice (2004) offered further ideas for special populations of patients, such as those with advanced disease, diminished functional abilities, and language barriers.

Symptom Clusters

Oncology nurses' knowledge of symptom clusters better assists nurses in targeting individual symptoms as well as the symptom within the cluster (Kim, McGuire, Tulman, & Barsevick, 2005). Symptom clusters are two, three, or more coexisting symptoms that are related but may be of differing etiologies and of varying time lengths (Esper & Heidrich, 2005; Kim et al.). Untreated or poorly treated symptom clusters may unfavorably affect patient outcomes and contribute to overall patient morbidity. Clinical experience has shown that older adults with cancer and patients of any age with advanced-stage disease could potentially experience greater symptomatology. A solid evidence base has emerged in this area, and multiple symptom cluster groupings have been proposed (Armstrong, Cohen, Eriksen, & Hickey, 2004; Bruera, Schmitz, Pither, Neumann, & Hanson, 2000; Dodd, Miaskowski, & Paul, 2001; Esper & Heidrich; Gift,

Jablonski, Stommel, & Given, 2004; Parker, Kimble, Dunbar, & Clark, 2005; So et al., 2009):

- Anxiety, agitation, and delirium
- Cough, breathlessness, and fatigue
- Dyspnea, anxiety, and fatigue
- Fatigue, depression, pain, menopausal symptoms, and sleep disturbances
- Fatigue, nausea, weakness, appetite loss, weight loss, altered taste, and vomiting
- Fatigue, pain, anxiety, and depression
- Nausea, anorexia, and dehydration
- Pain and depression
- Pain and fatigue
- Pain, constipation, and confusion
- Pain, fatigue, and sleep disturbances.

Application to Practice: Examples of Efficacy and Safety of CAM Therapies by Symptom

The popularity and availability of CAM therapies have enhanced conventional approaches to symptom management. Surveys, secondary analyses, systematic reviews, and studies support that CAM use is pervasive in symptom management and in palliative and end-of-life care (Fouladbakhsh, Stommel, Given, & Given, 2005; Lafferty, Downey, McCarty, Standish, & Patrick, 2006; Lengacher et al., 2006; Yates et al., 2005). Use, though, does not signify efficacy and safety. However, some CAM modalities can be safely used and have proven efficacy, and patients commonly use both conventional and CAM approaches to address signs and symptoms. For the sake of simplicity in this handbook, the "signs" and "symptoms" will be used under the umbrella of symptom management, recognizing that some may be separate medical conditions with their own diagnostic criteria (e.g., depression or insomnia). Efficacy and safety data from several reputable sources are reviewed in the following section for these symptoms:

- Anorexia-cachexia
- Anxiety
- Cognitive dysfunction
- Constipation
- Depression
- Diarrhea
- Fatigue
- Hormonal changes and hot flashes
- Insomnia
- Mucositis
- Myelosuppression
- Nausea and vomiting

- Nutritional issues
- Pain
- Sexual alterations
- Taste changes
- Xerostomia.

References

Armstrong, T.S., Cohen, M.Z., Eriksen, L.R., & Hickey, J.V. (2004). Symptom clusters in oncology patients and implications for symptom research in people with primary brain tumors. *Journal of Nursing Scholarship, 36*(3), 197–206.

Bruera, E., Schmitz, B., Pither, J., Neumann, C.M., & Hanson, J. (2000). The frequency and correlates of dyspnea in patients with advanced cancer. *Journal of Pain and Symptom Management, 19*(5), 357–362.

Dodd, M.J., Miaskowski, C., & Paul, S.M. (2001). Symptom clusters and their effect on the functional status of patients with cancer. *Oncology Nursing Forum, 28*(3), 465–470.

Eaton, L.H., & Tipton, J.M. (Eds.). (2009). *Putting evidence into practice: Improving oncology patient outcomes.* Pittsburgh, PA: Oncology Nursing Society.

Esper, P., & Heidrich, D. (2005). Symptom clusters in advanced illness. *Seminars in Oncology Nursing, 21*(1), 20–28.

Fouladbakhsh, J.M., Stommel, M., Given, B., & Given, C. (2005). Predictors of use of complementary and alternative therapies by cancer patients. *Oncology Nursing Forum, 32*(6), 1115–1123.

Gift, A.G., Jablonski, A., Stommel, M., & Given, C.W. (2004). Symptom clusters in elderly patients with lung cancer. *Oncology Nursing Forum, 31*(2), 202–212.

Kim, H.J., McGuire, D.B., Tulman, L., & Barsevick, A.M. (2005). Symptom clusters: Concept analysis and clinical implications for oncology nursing. *Cancer Nursing, 28*(4), 270–282.

Lafferty, W.E., Downey, L., McCarty, R.L., Standish, L.J., & Patrick, D.L. (2006). Evaluating CAM treatment at the end of life: A review of clinical trials for massage and meditation. *Complementary Therapies in Medicine, 14*(2), 100–112.

Lengacher, C.A., Bennet, M.P., Kip, K.E., Gonzalez, L., Jacobsen, P., & Cox, C.E. (2006). Relief of symptoms, side effects, and psychological distress through use of complementary and alternative medicine in women with breast cancer. *Oncology Nursing Forum, 33*(1), 97–104.

Paice, J. (2004). Assessment of symptom clusters in people with cancer. *Journal of the National Cancer Institute Monographs, 2004*(32), 98–102.

Parker, K.P., Kimble, L.P., Dunbar, S.B., & Clark, P.C. (2005). Symptom interactions as mechanisms underlying symptom pairs and clusters. *Journal of Nursing Scholarship, 37*(3), 209–215.

So, W.K., Marsh, G., Ling, W.M., Leung, F.Y., Lo, J.C., Yeung, M., et al. (2009). The symptom cluster of fatigue, pain, anxiety, and depression and the effect on the quality of life of women receiving treatment for breast cancer: A multicenter study [Online exclusive]. *Oncology Nursing Forum, 36*(4), E205–E214. Retrieved November 25, 2009, from http://ons.metapress.com/content/04g84475179605w8

Yarbro, C.H., Frogge, M.H., & Goodman, M. (Eds.). (2005). *Cancer nursing: Principles and practice* (6th ed.). Sudbury, MA: Jones and Bartlett.

Yates, J.S., Mustian, K.M., Morrow, G.R., Gillies, L.J., Padmanaban, D., Atkins, J.N., et al. (2005). Prevalence of complementary and alternative medicine use in cancer patients during treatment. *Supportive Care in Cancer, 13*(10), 806–811.

Anorexia-Cachexia Syndrome

Introduction

Anorexia is the loss of appetite or desire to eat. It may be a result of the cancer diagnosis or treatment. Anorexia can contribute to the course of cachexia, which is a progressive wasting syndrome that is not well understood. Anorexia-cachexia syndrome is characterized by a loss of appetite and weight, tissue wasting, and decreases in muscle mass and adipose tissue. Combinations of stomatitis, mucositis, taste alterations, xerostomia, infection, pain, dyspnea, and depression negatively contribute to this syndrome.

Toxicity grading for this symptom according to the NCI Cancer Therapy Evaluation Program (CTEP) Common Terminology Criteria for Adverse Events (CTCAE) can be added to the clinical evaluation and reported in the medical record. Currently, the adverse event is termed *anorexia*; anorexia-cachexia syndrome does not have a separate grading. The criteria range from loss of appetite (grade 1) to life-threatening consequences (grade 4) to death (grade 5) (NCI CTEP, 2009) (see Table 10).

Table 10. Common Terminology Criteria for Adverse Events: Metabolism and Nutrition Disorder

Adverse Event	Grade				
	1	2	3	4	5
Anorexia	Loss of appetite without alteration in eating foods	Oral intake altered without significant weight loss or malnutrition; oral nutritional supplements indicated	Associated with significant weight loss or malnutrition (e.g., inadequate oral caloric and/or fluid intake); tube feeding or TPN indicated	Life-threatening consequences; urgent intervention indicated	Death

TPN—total parenteral nutrition

Note. From *Common Terminology Criteria for Adverse Events* [v.4.02] (p. 44), by National Cancer Institute Cancer Therapy Evaluation Program, 2009. Retrieved November 23, 2009, from http://evs.nci.nih.gov/ftp1/CTCAE/CTCAE_4.02_2009-09-15_QuickReference_8.5x11.pdf.

Evidence for Practice

Successful conventional interventions are available to treat aspects of this syndrome as seen in *Putting Evidence Into Practice: Improving Oncology Patient Outcomes* (Adams, Cunningham, Caruso, Norling, & Shepard, 2009). Patients who choose to augment conventional approaches have economical, safe, and effective CAM therapy options.

Evidence	Natural Standard	Natural Medicines Comprehensive Database	Physician Data Query
Strong Scientific Evidence	• Vitamin A	• None at this time	• None at this time
Good to Moderate Scientific Evidence	• None at this time	• Branched-chain amino acids	• None at this time
Weak, Negative, or Conflicting Scientific Evidence	• Bee pollen • Dehydroepiandroster-one (DHEA) • Essiac • Hydrazine sulfate • Licorice • Melatonin • Soy supplements • Vitamin supplementation	• None at this time	• Cyproheptadine • Omega-3 fatty ac-ids

Examples of Ongoing Science

Cochrane Collaboration Systematic Reviews

• Eicosapentaenoic Acid (EPA, an Omega-3 Fatty Acid From Fish Oils) for the Treatment of Cancer Cachexia (Dewey, Baughan, Dean, Higgins, & Johnson, 2007)

Cochrane Collaboration Protocols

• None at this time

Complete systematic review and protocol information may be accessed at www.cochrane.org/index.htm.

Examples of Clinical Trials

- Megestrol Versus Eicosapentaenoic Acid-Enriched Nutritional Supplement Versus Both in Patients With Cancer-Related Cachexia and Anorexia (Phase III. Sponsor: NCI. Protocol IDs: NCCTG-989255, NCT00031707, NCI-P02-0205, CAN-NCIC-SC18. Closed.)
- Omega-3 Fatty Acids in Advanced Cancer Patients With Cachexia (Phase I/II. Sponsor: NCI. Protocol IDs: CLB-9473, NCT000003077, NCI-P97-0097. Closed.)

Complete clinical trial information may be accessed at http://cancer.gov/clinicaltrials.

Special Considerations

Pediatrics

The Children's Oncology Group (COG) Nutrition Committee is furthering the knowledge of nutrition in children with cancer by education and the conduct of clinical trials. COG has developed an algorithm as a guideline for nutritional intervention (Children's Hospital of New York-Presbyterian, 2009).

Older Adults

Anorexia may be secondary to dementia, depression, or malignancy in older adults. Visual or sensory deficits, living alone, low income, lack of transportation, or living in a group setting can predispose older adults to the development of malnutrition (American Geriatrics Society, 2009).

Summary

Anorexia-cachexia syndrome commonly occurs in patients with cancer. Nutritional considerations should focus on balanced nutrition, not just increased calories. Safe and effective CAM interventions are emerging with a scientific basis for incorporation into practice.

References

Adams, L.A., Cunningham, R.S., Caruso, R.A., Norling, M.J., & Shepard, N. (2009). ONS PEP resource: Anorexia. In L.H. Eaton & J.M. Tipton (Eds.), *Putting evidence into practice: Improving oncology patient outcomes* (pp. 31–36). Pittsburgh, PA: Oncology Nursing Society.
American Geriatrics Society. (2009). *Palliative care.* Retrieved August 20, 2009, from http://www.americangeriatrics.org

Children's Hospital of New York-Presbyterian. (2009). *The Integrative Therapies Program for Children With Cancer, 2009.* Retrieved August 20, 2009, from http://integrativetherapies.columbia.edu

Dewey, A., Baughan, C., Dean, T.P., Higgins, B., & Johnson, I. (2007). Eicosapentaenoic acid (EPA, an omega-3 fatty acid from fish oils) for the treatment of cancer cachexia. *Cochrane Database of Systematic Reviews* 2007, Issue 1. Art. No.: CD004597. DOI: 10.1002/14651858. CD004597.pub2

National Cancer Institute. (2009). *Nutrition in cancer care (PDQ®)* [Health professional version]. Retrieved August 20, 2009, from http://www.cancer.gov/cancertopics/pdq/supportivecare/nutrition/healthprofessional

National Cancer Institute Cancer Therapy Evaluation Program. (2009). *Common terminology criteria for adverse events* [v.4.02]. Retrieved August 20, 2009, from http://evs.nci.nih.gov/ftp1/CTCAE/CTCAE_4.02_2009-09-15_QuickReference_8.5x11.pdf

Natural Medicines Comprehensive Database. (n.d.). *Anorexia.* Retrieved August 20, 2009, from http://www.naturaldatabase.com

Natural Standard Database. (n.d.). *Cachexia (cancer related).* Retrieved August 20, 2009, from http://www.naturalstandard.com

Anxiety

Introduction

Anxiety is one of the most common psychological responses to the cancer experience. The American Psychological Association (n.d.) defines *anxiety* as an emotion characterized by feelings of tension, worried thoughts, and physical changes such as increased blood pressure. People with anxiety frequently have recurring intrusive thoughts and concerns and may have physical symptoms. Anxiety and depression are frequently seen concurrently in all age groups.

Patients who have shortness of breath, sweating, light-headedness, palpitations, intense fear, the inability to absorb information, or the inability to cooperate with medical procedures may be experiencing an anxiety disorder that was present before they became ill with cancer and that recurs because of the stress of the diagnosis and treatment. Patients with cancer can present with the following anxiety disorders: adjustment disorder, panic disorder, phobias, obsessive-compulsive disorder, post-traumatic stress disorder, generalized anxiety disorder, or anxiety disorder that is caused by other general medical conditions.

Toxicity grading for this symptom according to the CTCAE (NCI CTEP, 2009) can be added to the clinical assessment and reported in the medical record (see Table 11).

Adverse Event	Grade				
	1	2	3	4	5
Anxiety	Mild symptoms, intervention not indicated	Moderate symptoms; limiting instrumental ADL	Severe symptoms; limiting self-care ADL; hospitalization not indicated	Life threatening; hospitalization indicated	Death

Table 11. Common Terminology Criteria for Adverse Events: Anxiety (Psychiatric Disorders)

ADL—activities of daily living

Note. From *Common Terminology Criteria for Adverse Events* [v.4.02] (p. 57), by National Cancer Institute Cancer Therapy Evaluation Program, 2009. Retrieved November 23, 2009, from http://evs.nci.nih.gov/ftp1/CTCAE/CTCAE_4.02_2009-09-15_QuickReference_8.5x11.pdf.

Evidence for Practice

Safe and effective interventions are available to address anxiety as seen in *Putting Evidence Into Practice: Improving Oncology Patient Outcomes* (Swanson et al., 2009). The following CAM therapies have been evaluated for safety and efficacy.

Evidence	Natural Standard	Natural Medicines Comprehensive Database	Physician Data Query
Strong Scientific Evidence	• Kava • Music therapy	• None reported	• Directly confront problem • View situation as a problem to be solved or a challenge • Try to be flexible • Think of major events as series of step-by-step tasks • Use support and resources
Good to Moderate Scientific Evidence	• Art therapy • Chiropractic spinal manipulative therapy • Hypnosis • Meditation • Peppermint • Relaxation • Therapeutic touch • Yoga	• Possibly effective – Kava – Melatonin – Passion flower	• None reported
Weak, Negative, or Conflicting Scientific Evidence	• Conflicting – 5-hydroxy-L-tryptophan (5-HTP) – Acupressure, shiatsu – Acupuncture – Aromatherapy – Bach® (Nelsons) flower remedies – Bacopa – Black currant – Black tea – Borage seed oil – Bowen therapy – Gotu kola – Green tea – Guided imagery	• Insufficient evidence – 5-HTP – Aromatherapy – Autogenic training – Beer – Bergamot oil – California poppy – Ginkgo biloba – Hawthorn – Magnesium – Melatonin – Relaxation therapy – Roseroot	• None reported

(Continued on next page)

Evidence	Natural Standard	Natural Medicines Comprehensive Database	Physician Data Query
Weak, Negative, or Conflicting Scientific Evidence (cont.)	• Hawthorn • Healing touch • Kava • Lavender • Lemon balm • Massage • Meditation • Passion flower • Prayer, distant healing • Qigong • Reflexology • Rolfing® (Rolf Institute of Structural Integration)—structural integration • Rosemary • Sandalwood • St. John's wort • Sweet almond • Tai chi • Thymus extract • Valerian	− Skullcap − Theanine − Valerian − Wine − Yoga	
Strong Negative Evidence	• Trigger point therapy		

Examples of Ongoing Science

Cochrane Collaboration Systematic Reviews

• Kava Extract Versus Placebo for Treating Anxiety (Pittler & Ernst, 2003)

Cochrane Collaboration Protocols

• None at this time

Complete systematic review and protocol information may be accessed at www.cochrane.org/index.htm.

Examples of Clinical Trials

• Study of Anxiety Using the Memorial Anxiety Scale in African American Men With Prostate Cancer (No phase specified. Supportive care. Sponsor: NCI. Protocol IDs: MSKCC-07125, MSK IRB #07-125, NCT00602654. Active.)

- Anxiety and Depression Levels in Cancer Patients After Self Application of EFT (Emotional Freedom Techniques) (No phase specified. Supportive care. Sponsor: Pharmaceutical/industry. Protocol IDs: SMI-CHOL-82008, NCT00737399. Active.)

Complete clinical trial information may be accessed at http://cancer.gov/clinicaltrials.

Special Considerations

Pediatrics

Treatment of childhood cancer is a challenging, disruptive, and highly stressful experience for children and family. A general assumption is that children undergoing cancer treatment are at a higher risk for psychological distress, including depression and anxiety. Evidence to support this hypothesis is weak. Studies suggest that children treated for cancer and children who are long-term survivors of cancer experience few psychological adjustment problems. There is evidence that children experience distress during the cancer treatment process. Distress appears to be most significant early in therapy, typically when frequent hospitalizations are necessary, with a pattern of less distress occurring over time (Eiser, Hill, & Vance, 2000; Sawyer, Antoniou, Toogood, Rice, & Boghurt, 2000; Zebrack et al., 2004).

Older Adults

See Depression.

Summary

Anxiety is a normal reaction to cancer and may be experienced while undergoing a cancer screening or diagnostic test, waiting for test results, receiving a cancer diagnosis, during cancer treatment, or anticipating a cancer recurrence. Anxiety associated with cancer can increase pain, cause insomnia or nausea and vomiting, and interfere with quality of life. Feelings of anxiety increase or decrease at different times, and the level of anxiety experienced by one person may differ from that experienced by another. For patients with a history of an anxiety disorder that preceded their cancer diagnosis, anxiety can become overwhelming and have the potential to interfere with cancer treatment.

References

American Psychological Association. (n.d.). *Anxiety.* Retrieved December 22, 2009, from http://apa.org/topics/anxiety/index.aspx

Eiser, C., Hill, J.J., & Vance, Y.H. (2000). Examining the psychological consequences of surviving childhood cancer: Systematic review as a research method in pediatric psychology. *Journal of Pediatric Psychology, 25*(6), 449–460.

National Cancer Institute. (2009). *Supportive and palliative care: Anxiety disorder (PDQ®).* Retrieved August 20, 2009, from http://www.cancer.gov/cancertopics/pdq/supportivecare

National Cancer Institute Cancer Therapy Evaluation Program. (2009). *Common terminology criteria for adverse events* [v.4.02]. Retrieved August 20, 2009, from http://evs.nci.nih.gov/ftp1/CTCAE/CTCAE_4.02_2009-09-15_QuickReference_8.5x11.pdf.

Natural Medicines Comprehensive Database. (n.d.). *Natural medicines in the clinical management of anxiety.* Retrieved December 17, 2009, from http://www.naturaldatabase.com

Natural Standard Database. (n.d.). *Anxiety disorders.* Retrieved August 20, 2009, from http://www.naturalstandard.com

Pittler, M.H., & Ernst, E. (2003). Kava extract versus placebo for treating anxiety. *Cochrane Database of Systematic Reviews* 2003, Issue 1. Art. No.: CD003383. DOI: 10.1002/14651858.CD003383.

Sawyer, M., Antoniou, G., Toogood, I., Rice, M., & Boghurt, P. (2000). Childhood cancer: A 4-year prospective study of the psychological adjustment of children and parents. *Journal of Pediatric Hematology Oncology, 22*(3), 214–220.

Swanson, S.A., Sheldon, L.K., Dolce, A.H., Marsh, K., & Summers, J.A. (2009). ONS PEP resource: Anxiety. In L.H. Eaton & J.M. Tipton (Eds.), *Putting evidence into practice: Improving oncology patient outcomes* (pp. 43–50). Pittsburgh, PA: Oncology Nursing Society.

Zebrack, B.J., Gurney, J.G., Oeffinger, K,, Witton, J., Packer, R.J., Mertens, A., et al. (2004). Psychological outcomes in long-term survivors of childhood brain cancer: A report from the childhood cancer survivor study. *Journal of Clinical Oncology, 22*(6), 999–1006.

Cognitive Dysfunction

Introduction

Cognitive dysfunction or impairment is described as difficulty with thinking ability, including memory loss, distractibility, and difficulty with multitasking and arithmetic and language skills. Researchers note the difference between acute neurologic impairment and what is referred to as "chemo brain." The incidence of mild to moderate cognitive dysfunction related to chemotherapy to treat cancer has been confirmed by retrospective and prospective clinical trials (Jansen, Miaskowski, Dodd, Dowling, & Kramer, 2005; Myers, 2009).

With noted exceptions, standard doses of chemotherapy had not been reported to cross the blood-brain barrier (Ahles & Saykin, 2001; Saykin, Ahles, & McDonald, 2003). Wilkes and Barton-Burke (2007) noted that the exceptions included methotrexate, cisplatin, cytarabine, ifosfamide, procarbazine, temozolomide, carmustine, and lomustine, and Wong and Berkenblit (2004) added topotecan. Ahles and Saykin reported that higher-than-expected levels of chemotherapy were found in the brain and cerebral spinal fluid. This finding has led to further investigation to determine this as a possible cause of "chemo brain."

Toxicity grading for this symptom according to the CTCAE (NCI CTEP, 2009) is shown in Table 12.

Adverse Event	Grade				
	1	2	3	4	5
Cognitive disturbance	Mild cognitive disability; not interfering with work/school/life performance; specialized educational services/devices not indicated	Moderate cognitive disability; interfering with work/school/life performance but capable of independent living; specialized resources on part-time basis indicated	Severe cognitive disability; significant impairment of work/school/life performance	–	–

Table 12. Common Terminology Criteria for Adverse Events: Cognitive Disturbance

Note. From *Common Terminology Criteria for Adverse Events* [v.4.02] (p. 51), by National Cancer Institute Cancer Therapy Evaluation Program, 2009. Retrieved November 23, 2009, from http://evs.nci.nih.gov/ftp1/CTCAE/CTCAE_4.02_2009-09-15_QuickReference_8.5x11.pdf.

Evidence for Practice

Evidence	Natural Standard	Natural Medicines Comprehensive Database	Physician Data Query
Strong Scientific Evidence	• None at this time	• None at this time	• None at this time
Good to Moderate Scientific Evidence	• None at this time	• None at this time	• None at this time
Weak, Negative, or Conflicting Scientific Evidence	• In a study conducted at West Virginia School of Medicine, one group of rats received two common cancer drugs, doxorubicin (Adriamycin®, Bedford Laboratories) and cyclophosphamide (Cytoxan®, Bristol-Myers Squibb Co.), four times weekly. Compared to the control animals, the rats that received chemotherapy had lower memory scores, indicating "chemo brain." However, "chemo brain" was prevented when rats received antioxidant N-acetyl cysteine injections three times weekly during chemotherapy.	• None at this time	• None

Examples of Ongoing Science

Cochrane Collaboration Systematic Reviews

• None at this time

Cochrane Collaboration Protocols

• None at this time

Complete systematic review and protocol information may be accessed at www.cochrane.org/index.htm.

Examples of Clinical Trials

- Assessment and Rehabilitation of Cognitive Impairments in Pediatric Survivors of Cancer Age 9–16 (No phase specified. Sponsor: NCI. Protocol IDs: PEDSVAR0003, 97817, NCT00490334, PedsVar0003, NCT00490334. Active as of September 1, 2009.)
- Exercise and Cognitive-Psychosocial Functions in Men With Prostate Cancer Receiving Androgen Depletion Therapy. Age 50 and Over. (No phase specified. Sponsor: NCI. Protocol IDs: H2008:318, NCT00856102. Approved but not active as of September 1, 2009.)

Complete clinical trial information may be accessed at http://cancer.gov/clinicaltrials.

Special Considerations

Pediatrics

Although more is known about "chemo brain," there remains much to be learned concerning cognitive dysfunction and impairment and CAM therapies for pediatric cancer survivors.

Older Adults

Changes in cognition were long thought to be an inevitable consequence of cancer treatment. Clinicians have much to learn about CAM therapies for cognitive impairment in older patients.

Summary

Research is needed to identify patients who are vulnerable to cognitive dysfunction from chemotherapy and the CAM therapies most likely to support traditional therapies in the prevention of or rehabilitation from cognitive dysfunction.

References

Ahles, T.A., & Saykin, A.J. (2001). Cognitive effects of standard-dose chemotherapy in patients with cancer. *Cancer Investigation, 19*(8), 812–820.

Jansen, C., Miaskowski, C., Dodd, M., Dowling, G., & Kramer, J. (2005). Potential mechanisms for chemotherapy-induced impairments in cognitive function. *Oncology Nursing Forum, 32*(6), 1151–1163.

Myers, J. (2009). A comparison of the theory of unpleasant symptoms and the conceptual model of chemotherapy-related changes in cognitive function [Online exclusive]. *Oncology Nursing Forum, 36*(1), E1–E9. Retrieved November 18, 2009, from http://ons.metapress.com/content/l00222q316231931

National Cancer Institute. (2009). *Complementary and alternative medicine in cancer treatment (PDQ®)* [Patient version]. Retrieved August 20, 2009, from http://www.cancer.gov/cancertopics/pdq/cam/cam-cancer-treatment

National Cancer Institute Cancer Therapy Evaluation Program. (2009). *Common terminology criteria for adverse events* [v.4.02]. Retrieved August 20, 2009, from http://evs.nci.nih.gov/ftp1/CTCAE/CTCAE_4.02_2009-09-15_QuickReference_8.5x11.pdf

Natural Medicines Comprehensive Database. (n.d.). *Cognitive function.* Retrieved December 17, 2009, from http://www.naturaldatabase.com

Natural Standard Database. (n.d.). *Cognitive deficits.* Retrieved December 17, 2009, from http://www.naturalstandard.com

Saykin, A.J., Ahles, T.A., & McDonald, B.C. (2003). Mechanisms of chemotherapy-induced cognitive disorders: Neuropsychological, pathophysiological, and neuroimaging perspectives. *Seminars in Clinical Neuropsychiatry, 8*(4), 201–216.

Wilkes, G.M., & Barton-Burke, M. (2007). *Oncology nursing drug handbook.* Sudbury, MA: Jones and Bartlett.

Wong, E.T., & Berkenblit, A. (2004). The role of topotecan in the treatment of brain metastases. *Oncologist, 9*(1), 68–79.

Constipation

Introduction

Constipation is a disorder characterized by the irregular and infrequent or difficult evacuation of the bowels (NCI, 2009). Cancer-related causes of constipation are mechanical pressure on the bowel (e.g., tumor, ascites), medications (e.g., chemotherapy, opioids), interrupted neural transmission of the desire to defecate (e.g., pressure on the spinal cord), hypercalcemia, brachytherapy (gynecologic or prostate cancer), and depression. Other causative factors may include anorexia-cachexia syndrome, dysphagia, mucositis, or poorly controlled nausea and vomiting.

Toxicity grading for this symptom according to the CTCAE (NCI CTEP, 2009) can be added to the clinical evaluation and reported in the medical record. The criteria range from occasional or intermittent symptoms (grade 1) to life-threatening consequences (grade 4) to death (grade 5) (see Table 13).

Table 13. Common Terminology Criteria for Adverse Events: Gastrointestinal Disorders—Constipation

Adverse Event	Grade				
	1	2	3	4	5
Constipation	Occasional or intermittent symptoms; occasional use of stool softeners, laxatives, dietary modification, or enema	Persistent symptoms with regular use of laxative or enemas; limiting instrumental ADL	Obstipation with manual evacuation indicated; limiting self-care ADL	Life-threatening consequences; urgent intervention indicated	Death

ADL—activities of daily living

Note. From *Common Terminology Criteria for Adverse Events* [v.4.02] (p. 32), by National Cancer Institute Cancer Therapy Evaluation Program, 2009. Retrieved November 23, 2009, from http://evs.nci.nih .gov/ftp1/CTCAE/CTCAE_4.02_2009-09-15_QuickReference_8.5x11.pdf.

Evidence for Practice

Successful conventional interventions are available to treat aspects of this condition as seen in *Putting Evidence Into Practice: Improving Oncology Patient Outcomes* (Bisanz et al., 2009). Patients who choose to augment conventional approaches have several economical, safe, and effective CAM nutritional therapy options available and potential future options.

Evidence	Natural Standard	Natural Medicines Comprehensive Database	Physician Data Query
Strong Scientific Evidence	• Phosphates, phosphorus	• Black psyllium • Blond psyllium • Magnesium	• Psyllium • Magnesium • Sodium phosphate
Good to Moderate Scientific Evidence	• Aloe • Psyllium	• Cascara • European buckthorn • Glycerol • Olive • Senna	• None at this time
Weak, Negative, or Conflicting Scientific Evidence	• Ayurveda (Misrakasneham) • Barley • Cascara sagrada • Flaxseed • Iodine • Probiotics	• Alder buckthorn • Aloe	• None at this time

Examples of Ongoing Science

Cochrane Collaboration Systematic Reviews

• Laxatives for the Management of Constipation in Palliative Care Patients (Miles, Fellowes, Goodman, & Wilkinson, 2006)

Cochrane Collaboration Protocols

• Acupuncture for Chronic Constipation (Zhao, Liu, Liu, & Peng, 2003)
    Complete systematic review and protocol information may be accessed at www.cochrane.org/index.htm.

Examples of Clinical Trials

• Study Evaluating Safety and Efficacy of Subcutaneous Methylnaltrexone on Opioid-Induced Constipation in Cancer Subjects (Phase IV. Supportive care. Protocol IDs: 3200K1-4006, NCT00858754. Active.)

- Acupuncture to Prevent Postoperative Bowel Paralysis (Paralytic Ileus) (Phase II. Supportive care. Protocol IDs: R21 AT0011065-01A1, NCT00065234. Closed.)

Complete clinical trial information may be accessed at http://cancer.gov/clinicaltrials.

Special Considerations

Pediatrics

The COG Nutrition Committee is furthering the knowledge of nutrition in children with cancer by education and the conduct of clinical trials. COG has developed an algorithm as a guideline for nutritional intervention (Children's Hospital of New York-Presbyterian, 2009).

Older Adults

About 30% of adults aged 65 years or older have chronic constipation, with a greater incidence noted in women. Constipation may occur as a side effect of drugs or may be a manifestation of metabolic or neurologic disease. In all situations, colonic obstruction must be excluded. Constipation among patients with dementia is common, especially with the use of psychotropic medications. A proactive approach is recommended, as patients may not always be relied upon to describe symptoms (National Institute on Aging, 2009).

Summary

Constipation commonly occurs in patients with cancer. Conventional interventions ameliorating this symptom are safe and effective. CAM interventions are emerging with a supportive scientific basis for incorporation into practice.

References

Bisanz, A.K., Woolery, M.J., Lyons, H.F., Gaido, L., Yenulevich, M., & Fulton, S. (2009). ONS PEP resource: Constipation. In L.H. Eaton & J.M. Tipton (Eds.), *Putting evidence into practice: Improving oncology patient outcomes* (pp. 93–104). Pittsburgh, PA: Oncology Nursing Society.

Children's Hospital of New York-Presbyterian. (2009). *The Integrative Therapies Program for Children With Cancer, 2009.* Retrieved August 20, 2009, from http://integrativetherapies.columbia.edu

Miles, C., Fellowes, D., Goodman, M.L., & Wilkinson, S.S.M. (2006, October). Laxatives for the management of constipation in palliative care patients. *Cochrane Database of Systematic*

Reviews, 2006, Issue 4. Art. No.: CD003448. DOI: 10.1002/14651858.CD003448.pub2. Retrieved November 17, 2009, from http://www.cochrane.org/reviews/en/ab003448.html

National Cancer Institute. (2009, October). *Gastrointestinal complications (PDQ®): Constipation* [Health professional version]. Retrieved November 17, 2009, from http://www.cancer.gov/cancertopics/pdq/supportivecare/gastrointestinalcomplications/HealthProfessional/page3

National Cancer Institute Cancer Therapy Evaluation Program. (2009). *Common terminology criteria for adverse events* [v.4.02]. Retrieved August 20, 2009, from http://evs.nci.nih.gov/ftp1/CTCAE/CTCAE_4.02_2009-09-15_QuickReference_8.5x11.pdf

National Institute on Aging. (2009, December). *Age Page: Concerned about constipation?* Retrieved December 21, 2009, from http://www.nia.nih.gov/HealthInformation/Publications/constipation.htm

Natural Medicines Comprehensive Database. (n.d.). *Constipation.* Retrieved August 20, 2009, from http://www.naturaldatabase.com

Natural Standard Database. (n.d.). *Constipation (cancer related).* Retrieved August 20, 2009, from http://www.naturalstandard.com

Zhao, H., Liu, J.P., Liu, Z., & Peng, W. (2003). Acupuncture for chronic constipation (Protocol). *Cochrane Database of Systematic Reviews* 2003, Issue 2. Art. No.: CD004117. DOI: 10.1002/14651858.CD004117.

Depression

Introduction

Depression or depressive disorder is an illness that involves the body, mood, and thoughts. Depression is considered a mood disorder. Imbalances in the brain chemicals serotonin, norepinephrine, and dopamine are linked to depression. Depression affects the way a person eats and sleeps, the way one feels about oneself, and the way one thinks about life situations. Depression is different than the passing emotional experience of sadness; it is persistent and can significantly interfere with an individual's thoughts, behavior, mood, activity, and physical health.

The incidence of depression in people with cancer is considerably higher than in the general population. Depression is considered a comorbid disabling syndrome that affects approximately 15%–25% of patients with cancer and is believed to affect men and women with cancer equally (Martin & Jackson, 2000). Individuals and families who face a cancer diagnosis will experience varying levels of stress and emotional upset. Depression in patients with cancer has a major negative impact on their families.

According to the American Psychiatric Association's *Diagnostic and Statistical Manual of Mental Disorders* (2000), symptoms that could indicate depression if they are present for more than two weeks include depressed mood, noticeably diminished interest or pleasure in activities that formerly were enjoyed, disturbances in eating and sleeping, social withdrawal, loss of energy, feelings of worthlessness or guilt, diminished ability to think, diminished ability to concentrate, and recurrent thoughts of death or suicide.

Toxicity grading for this symptom according to the CTCAE (NCI CTEP, 2009) can be added to the clinical assessment and reported in the medical record (see Table 14).

Evidence for Practice

Safe and effective interventions are available to address depression as seen in *Putting Evidence Into Practice: Improving Oncology Patient Outcomes* (Fulcher, Badger, Gunter, Marrs, & Reese, 2009). The following CAM therapies have been evaluated for safety and efficacy.

Table 14. Common Terminology Criteria for Adverse Events: Depression (Psychiatric Disorders)

Adverse Event	Grade				
	1	2	3	4	5
Depression	Mild depressive symptoms	Moderate depressive symptoms; limiting instrumental ADL	Severe depressive symptoms; limiting self-care ADL; hospitalization not indicated	Life-threatening consequences, threats of harm to self or others, hospitalization indicated	Death

ADL—activities of daily living

Note. From *Common Terminology Criteria for Adverse Events* [v.4.02] (p. 57), by National Cancer Institute Cancer Therapy Evaluation Program, 2009. Retrieved November 23, 2009, from http://evs.nci.nih.gov/ftp1/CTCAE/CTCAE_4.02_2009-09-15_QuickReference_8.5x11.pdf.

Evidence	Natural Standard	Natural Medicines Comprehensive Database	Physician Data Query
Strong Scientific Evidence	• Music therapy • Sage • St. John's wort (mild to moderate depression)	• Likely effective – SAMe – St. John's wort	• None reported
Good to Moderate Scientific Evidence	• Art therapy • 5-HTP • DHEA • Hypnosis, hypnotherapy • Phenylalanine • Yoga	• Possibly effective – 5-HTP – EPA – Fish oil – Folic acid – Saffron – Yoga	• None reported
Weak, Negative, or Conflicting Scientific Evidence	• Acupressure, shiatsu • Acupuncture • Ayurveda • Aromatherapy • Bach flower remedies • Chasteberry • Coleus • Creatine • Folate • Feldenkrais® (Feldenkrais Guild® of North America)	• Insufficient evidence – Acetyl L-carnitine – Acupuncture – Aromatherapy – Biofeedback – Chromium – DHEA – L-tryptophan – Phosphatidyl serine – Qigong	• St. John's wort for major depression

(Continued on next page)

Evidence	Natural Standard	Natural Medicines Comprehensive Database	Physician Data Query

Weak, Negative, or Conflicting Scientific Evidence (cont.)	• Ginkgo biloba
	• Ginseng
	• Guarana
	• Healing touch
	• Lavender
	• L-carnitine
	• Massage
	• Meditation
	• Melatonin
	• Omega-3 fish oils, fish oil, alpha-linolenic acid
	• Prayer, distant healing
	• Qigong
	• Reflexology
	• Reiki
	• Riboflavin (vitamin B_2)
	• SAMe
	• Tai chi
	• Therapeutic touch
	• Valerian
	• Vitamin B_6
	• Vitamin D
		• Possibly ineffective
		  – Inositol
		  – Melatonin
		  – Tyrosine	

Examples of Ongoing Science

Cochrane Collaboration Systematic Reviews

• Aromatherapy and Massage for Symptom Relief in Patients With Cancer (Fellowes, Barnes, & Wilkinson, 2008)

Cochrane Collaboration Protocols

• Psychosocial Interventions to Improve Quality of Life and Emotional Well-being for Recently Diagnosed Cancer Patients (Galway et al., 2008)

   Complete systematic review and protocol information may be accessed at www.cochrane.org/index.htm

Examples of Clinical Trials

• Depression Treatment and Screening in Ovarian Cancer Patients (Phase I. Supportive care. Sponsor: NCI, Other. Protocol IDs: ID02-258, NCT00515372. Active.)

- Study of Computerized Symptom Assessment and Classification of Pain, Depression, and Physical Function in Patients With Metastatic and/or Advanced Locoregional Cancer (No phase specified. Supportive care. Sponsor: Other. Protocol IDs: NUST-EPCRC-CSA, EPCRC-CSA, EU-20962. Active.)
- A collaborative-care, multidisciplinary intervention to treat depression in patients with cancer was more effective than usual care in relieving symptoms of depression in a study conducted at a community-based center serving a predominantly low-income Hispanic population. At 12 months, patients receiving the collaborative-care intervention also had significantly better social, emotional, and functional well-being (Ell et al., 2008).

Complete clinical trial information may be accessed at http://cancer.gov/clinicaltrials.

Special Considerations

Pediatrics

Information is limited concerning the incidence of depression in healthy children. Studies have estimated that 1.9% (age 7–12 in general pediatric practice) to 38% (in general practice) had problems that required major intervention by a psychiatrist (NCI, 2009). Teachers have estimated that as many as 10%–15% of their students are depressed. The Joint Commission on Mental Health of Children states that 1.4 million children younger than 18 years old need immediate help for disorders such as depression, but only one-third receive help (NCI).

Most children cope with the emotional upheaval related to cancer and demonstrate not only evidence of adaptation but positive psychosocial growth and development (NCI, 2009). A minority of children develop psychological problems including depression, anxiety, sleep disturbances, difficulties in interpersonal relationships, and noncompliance with treatment. These children require referral and intervention by a mental health specialist.

Older Adults

The incidence of depression is known to increase with age and has been associated with increased morbidities. Decker (2006) reported that depression is one of the most frequent reasons for seeking CAM therapies, including St. John's wort, autogenic training, music therapy, massage, exercise, aromatherapy, dance and movement therapy, and relaxation.

Summary

Incidence of depression is increased in people with cancer and their families. The incidence of depression increases with age. People with cancer will seek CAM therapies to assist in coping with depression. Assessment for depression, including use of CAM therapies, is needed throughout the cancer experience.

References

American Psychiatric Association. (2000). *Diagnostic and statistical manual of mental disorders* (4th ed., text rev.). Retrieved December 17, 2009, from http://www.psych.org/Main/Menu/Research/DSMIV/DSMIVTR.aspx

Decker, G. (2006). Complementary and alternative therapies. In D.G. Cope & A.M. Reb (Eds.), *An evidence-based approach to the treatment and care of the older adult with cancer* (pp. 485–528). Pittsburgh, PA: Oncology Nursing Society.

Ell, K., Xie, B., Quon, B., Quinn, D.I., Dwight-Johnson, M., & Lee, P.J. (2008). Randomized controlled trial of collaborative care management of depression among low-income patients with cancer. *Journal of Clinical Oncology, 26*(27), 4488–4496.

Fellowes, D., Barnes, K., & Wilkinson, S.S.M. (2008). Aromatherapy and massage for symptom relief in patients with cancer. *Cochrane Database of Systematic Reviews* 2008, Issue 4. Art. No.: CD002287. DOI: 10.1002/14651858.CD002287.pub3.

Fulcher, C.D., Badger, T.A., Gunter, A.K., Marrs, J.A., & Reese, J.M. (2009). ONS PEP resource: Depression. In L.H. Eaton & J.M. Tipton (Eds.), *Putting evidence into practice: Improving oncology patient outcomes* (pp. 111–118). Pittsburgh, PA: Oncology Nursing Society.

Galway, K., Black, A., Cantwell, M., Cardwell, C.R., Mills, M., & Donnelly, M. (2008). Psychosocial interventions to improve quality of life and emotional wellbeing for recently diagnosed cancer patients (Protocol). *Cochrane Database of Systematic Reviews* 2008, Issue 2. Art. No.: CD007064. DOI: 10.1002/14651858.CD007064.

Martin, A.C., & Jackson, K.C. (2000). Depression in palliative care patients. *Journal of Pharmaceutical Care in Pain and Symptom Control, 7*(4), 71–89.

National Cancer Institute. (2009). *Depression (PDQ®)* [Health professional version]. Retrieved November 23, 2009, from http://www.cancer.gov/cancertopics/pdq/supportivecare/depression/HealthProfessional/page7

National Cancer Institute Cancer Therapy Evaluation Program. (2009). *Common terminology criteria for adverse events* [v.4.02]. Retrieved August 20, 2009, from http://evs.nci.nih.gov/ftp1/CTCAE/CTCAE_4.02_2009-09-15_QuickReference_8.5x11.pdf

Natural Medicines Comprehensive Database. (n.d.). *Depression.* Retrieved December 17, 2009, from http://www.naturaldatabase.com

Natural Standard Database. (n.d.). *Depression.* Retrieved August 20, 2009, from http://www.naturalstandard.com

Diarrhea

Introduction

Diarrhea is a disorder characterized by frequent and watery bowel movements (NCI, 2009). Most cases of acute diarrhea have an abrupt onset, last one to two weeks in duration, have an infectious cause, and are self-limiting (Smart, 2003). Severe and uncontrolled diarrhea can lead to skin alterations with secondary infections, dehydration, electrolyte imbalance, and renal acid-base balance alterations. Cancer-related causes of diarrhea can be disease-related or treatment-related. Examples of disease-related causes are certain tumors (gastrinoma, vasoactive intestinal peptide tumor, carcinoid, lymphoma, and colorectal), colitis, enzyme insufficiency, or infectious processes (e.g., *Clostridium difficile*, cytomegalovirus). Examples of treatment-related causes are certain surgical procedures (colon resection, gastrectomy), chemotherapeutic agents, radiation to the abdomen or pelvis, or supportive care interventions (enteral feedings, antibiotics).

Toxicity grading for this symptom according to the CTCAE (NCI CTEP, 2009) can be added to the clinical evaluation and reported in the medical record. The criteria range from mild increase in number of stools or ostomy output (grade 1) to life-threatening consequences (grade 4) to death (grade 5) (see Table 15).

Table 15. Common Terminology Criteria for Adverse Events: Gastrointestinal Disorders—Diarrhea

Adverse Event	Grade				
	1	2	3	4	5
Diarrhea	Increase of < 4 stools per day over baseline; mild increase in ostomy output	Increase of 4–6 stools per day over baseline; moderate increase in	Increase of ≥ 7 stools per day over baseline; incontinence; hospitalization indicated;	Life-threatening consequences; urgent intervention indicated	Death

(Continued on next page)

Table 15. Common Terminology Criteria for Adverse Events: Gastrointestinal Disorders—Diarrhea *(Continued)*					
Adverse Event	**Grade**				
	1	**2**	**3**	**4**	**5**
	compared to baseline	ostomy output compared to baseline	severe increase in ostomy output compared to baseline; limiting self-care ADL		

ADL—activities of daily living

Note. From *Common Terminology Criteria for Adverse Events* [v.4.02] (p. 13), by National Cancer Institute Cancer Therapy Evaluation Program, 2009. Retrieved November 23, 2009, from http://evs.nci.nih.gov/ftp1/CTCAE/CTCAE_4.02_2009-09-15_QuickReference_8.5x11.pdf.

Evidence for Practice

Successful conventional interventions are available to treat aspects of this condition as seen in *Putting Evidence Into Practice: Improving Oncology Patient Outcomes* (Muehlbauer et al., 2009). Patients who choose to augment conventional approaches have several economical, safe, and effective CAM nutritional therapy options available.

Evidence	Natural Standard	Natural Medicines Comprehensive Database	Physician Data Query
Strong Scientific Evidence	• *Saccharomyces boulardii* (concurrent use with antibiotic therapy)	• None at this time	• None at this time
Good to Moderate Scientific Evidence	• Probiotics (*Lactobacillus*) • Psyllium • Soy	• *Lactobacillus* (for rotaviral diarrhea) • Zinc	• Probiotic functional foods
Weak, Negative, or Conflicting Scientific Evidence	• Arnica • Arrowroot • Berberine • Bilberry • Carob • Chamomile • Goldenseal • Slippery elm • Soy	• *Lactobacillus* (for antibiotic-associated, chemotherapy-induced)	• Glutamine

Examples of Ongoing Science

Cochrane Collaboration Systematic Reviews

- Probiotics for the Prevention of Pediatric Antibiotic-Associated Diarrhea (Johnston, Supina, Ospina, & Vohra, 2007)

Cochrane Collaboration Protocols

- Probiotics for the Prevention of *Clostridium Difficile* Associated Diarrhea in Adults and Children (Johnston & Thorlund, 2009)
  Complete systematic review and protocol information may be accessed at www.cochrane.org/index.htm.

Examples of Clinical Trials

- Study of Glutamine as Prophylaxis for Irinotecan Induced Diarrhea (Phase II. Supportive care. Sponsor: Alberta Cancer Board. Protocol IDs: GI-05-0024, NCT00255229. Open.)
- Lactobacillus Rhamnosus in Prevention of Chemotherapy-Related Diarrhea (Phase II. Supportive care, treatments. Sponsor: Helsinki University. Protocol IDs: ML 18581, NCT00197873. Open.)
  Complete clinical trial information may be accessed at http://cancer.gov/clinicaltrials.

Special Considerations

Pediatrics

The COG Nutrition Committee is furthering the knowledge of nutrition in children with cancer by education and the conduct of clinical trials. COG has developed an algorithm as a guideline for nutritional intervention (Children's Hospital of New York-Presbyterian, 2009).

Older Adults

Additional causes of diarrhea may be fecal impaction, lactose intolerance, and comorbid gastrointestinal (GI) conditions (e.g., irritable bowel syndrome, malabsorption, inflammatory bowel disease), infections, or medications (American Geriatrics Society, 2009). An increased risk for complications associated with diarrhea, such as dehydration, altered drug metabolism, compromised cardiac status, and confusion, exists within this population (Gardner & Cope, 2006).

Summary

Diarrhea commonly occurs in patients with cancer. Conventional interventions ameliorating this symptom are safe and effective. CAM interventions are emerging with a supportive scientific basis for incorporation into practice.

References

American Geriatrics Society. (2009). *Palliative care.* Retrieved August 20, 2009, from http://www.americangeriatrics.org

Children's Hospital of New York-Presbyterian. (2009). *Integrative Therapies Program for Children With Cancer, 2009.* Retrieved August 20, 2009, from http://integrativetherapies.columbia.edu

Gardner, N.M., & Cope, D.G. (2006). Symptom management of diarrhea and constipation. In D.G. Cope, & A.M. Reb (Eds.), *An evidence-based approach to the treatment and care of the older adult with cancer* (pp. 367–389). Pittsburgh, PA: Oncology Nursing Society.

Johnston, B.C., Supina, A.L., Ospina, M., & Vohra, S. (2007). Probiotics for the prevention of pediatric antibiotic-associated diarrhea. *Cochrane Database of Systematic Reviews* 2007, Issue 2. Art. No.: CD004827. DOI: 10.1002/14651858.CD004827.pub2.

Johnston, B.C., & Thorlund, K. (2009). Probiotics for the prevention of Clostridium difficile associated diarrhea in adults and children (Protocol). *Cochrane Database of Systematic Reviews* 2009, Issue 1. Art. No.: CD006095. DOI: 10.1002/14651858.CD006095.pub2.

Muehlbauer, P., Thorpe, D., Davis, A.B., Drabot, R.C., Kiker, E.S., & Rawlings, B.L. (2009). ONS PEP resource: Diarrhea. In L.H. Eaton & J.M. Tipton (Eds.), *Putting evidence into practice: Improving oncology patient outcomes* (pp. 125–134). Pittsburgh, PA: Oncology Nursing Society.

National Cancer Institute. (2009). *Gastrointestinal complications (PDQ®): Diarrhea* [Health professional version]. Retrieved August 20, 2009, from http://www.cancer.gov/cancertopics/pdq/supportivecare/gastrointestinalcomplications/HealthProfessional/page6

National Cancer Institute Cancer Therapy Evaluation Program. (2009). *Common terminology criteria for adverse events* [v.4.02]. Retrieved August 20, 2009, from http://evs.nci.nih.gov/ftp1/CTCAE/CTCAE_4.02_2009-09-15_QuickReference_8.5x11.pdf

Natural Medicines Comprehensive Database. (n.d.). *Diarrhea.* Retrieved August 20, 2009, from http://www.naturaldatabase.com

Natural Standard Database. (n.d.). *Diarrhea (cancer-related).* Retrieved August 20, 2009, from http://www.naturalstandard.com

Smart, S.R. (2003). Diarrhea. In T.M. Buttaro, J. Trybulski, P.P. Bailey, & J. Sandberg-Cook (Eds.), *Primary care: A collaborative practice* (2nd ed., pp. 652–654). St. Louis, MO: Mosby.

Fatigue

Introduction

Cancer-related fatigue has been defined as "a distressing, persistent, subjective sense of physical, emotional, and/or cognitive tiredness or exhaustion related to cancer or cancer treatment that is not proportional to recent activity and interferes with usual functioning" (National Comprehensive Cancer Network, 2009, p. FT-1). Cancer-related fatigue is the most common symptom reported by patients during cancer treatment (Lawrence, Kupelnick, Miller, Devine, & Lau, 2004). It may occur alone or clustered with other symptoms.

Fatigue is a subjective assessment and therefore self-report can provide an accurate assessment. Key to any assessment is to measure and compare the symptom at different times. Physiologic, treatable causes of fatigue, such as anemia, must be identified and addressed. Fatigue cannot be viewed as an inevitable consequence of cancer or cancer therapy to be tolerated.

Toxicity grading for this symptom according to the CTCAE (NCI CTEP, 2009) can be added to the clinical assessment and reported in the medical record (see Table 16).

Adverse Event	Grade				
	1	2	3	4	5
Fatigue	Fatigue relieved by rest	Fatigue not relieved by rest; limiting instrumental ADL	Fatigue not relieved by rest; limiting self-care ADL	–	–

Table 16. Common Terminology Criteria for Adverse Events: Fatigue (General Disorders and Administration Site Conditions)

ADL—activities of daily living

Note. From *Common Terminology Criteria for Adverse Events* [v.4.02] (p. 22), by National Cancer Institute Cancer Therapy Evaluation Program, 2009. Retrieved November 23, 2009, from http://evs.nci.nih.gov/ftp1/CTCAE/CTCAE_4.02_2009-09-15_QuickReference_8.5x11.pdf.

Evidence for Practice

Safe and effective conventional and CAM therapy interventions are available to address this syndrome as seen in Putting *Evidence Into Practice: Improving Oncology Patient Outcomes* (Mitchell, Beck, Hood, Moore, & Tanner, 2009). The following CAM therapies have been evaluated for safety and efficacy.

Evidence	Natural Standard	Natural Medicines Comprehensive Database	Physician Data Query
Strong Scientific Evidence	• None reported	• None reported	• None reported
Good to Moderate Scientific Evidence	• Probiotics (*Lactobacillus*) • Polarity therapy for radiation therapy–related fatigue • Exercise for men with prostate cancer receiving hormonal or radiation therapy • Ginseng for cancer-related fatigue • Psyllium • Soy	• None reported	• Exercise
Weak, Negative, or Conflicting Scientific Evidence	• DHEA • Reiki • Yoga • Acupuncture • Reflexology	• Acupressure • Possibly ineffective—none reported	• Exercise for fatigue in terminally ill patients

Examples of Ongoing Science

Cochrane Collaboration Systematic Reviews

• Exercise for the Management of Cancer-Related Fatigue in Adults (Cramp & Daniel, 2008)

Cochrane Collaboration Protocols

• Educational Interventions for the Management of Cancer-Related Fatigue in Adults (Bennett et al., 2009)

Complete systematic review and protocol information may be accessed at www.cochrane.org/index.htm.

Examples of Clinical Trials

- Fatigue Intervention Trial for Breast Cancer Survivors (Phase III. Supportive care. Sponsor: Other. Protocol IDs: MMC2007-46, NCT00513136. Active.)
- Phase III Randomized Study of American Ginseng in Patients With Cancer-Related Fatigue (Phase III. Supportive care. Sponsor: NCI. Protocol IDs: NCCTG-N07C2, N07C2, NCT00719563. Active.)

Complete clinical trial information may be accessed at http://cancer.gov/clinicaltrials.

Special Considerations

Pediatrics

Fatigue in children and adolescents with cancer has eluded definition, measurement, and intervention. Fatigue in these patients exists within a greater context of illness, treatment, and development.

Older Adults

Fatigue in older patients with cancer has not been well studied. Variables such as treatment, medical age of the patient, and the presence or absence of comorbidities affect fatigue in this population.

Summary

The etiology and mechanisms regarding fatigue in patients with cancer have not been determined, and practice patterns regarding management vary. The focus of medical management often is on identifying specific and potentially reversible correlated symptoms (e.g., anemia). Much of the information regarding interventions for fatigue relates either to healthy subjects or to fatigue as secondary to treatment-related anemia. Some recommendations for the management of fatigue in patients with cancer have been made, but with the exception of exercise, these are mostly theoretical and have not been the focus of scientific evaluation until recently.

References

Bennett, S., Purcell, A., Meredith, P., Beller, E., Haines, T., & Fleming, J. (2009). Educational interventions for the management of cancer-related fatigue in adults. *Cochrane Database of Systematic Reviews* 2009, Issue 4. Art. No.: CD008144. DOI: 10.1002/14651858 .CD008144.

Cramp, F., & Daniel, J. (2008). Exercise for the management of cancer-related fatigue in adults. *Cochrane Database of Systematic Reviews* 2008, Issue 2. Art. No.: CD006145. DOI: 10.1002/14651858.CD006145.pub2.

Lawrence, D.P., Kupelnick, D., Miller, K., Devine, D., & Lau, J. (2004). Evidence report on the occurrence, assessment, and treatment of fatigue in cancer patients. *Journal of the National Cancer Institute Monographs, 2004*(32), 40–50.

Mitchell, S.A., Beck, S.L., Hood, L.E., Moore, K., & Tanner, E.R. (2009). ONS PEP resource: Fatigue. In L.H. Eaton & J.M. Tipton (Eds.), *Putting evidence into practice: Improving oncology patient outcomes* (pp. 155–174). Pittsburgh, PA: Oncology Nursing Society.

National Cancer Institute. (2009, May). *Fatigue (PDQ®)*. Retrieved August 20, 2009, from http://www.cancer.gov/cancertopics/pdq/supportivecare/fatigue/healthprofessional

National Cancer Institute Cancer Therapy Evaluation Program. (2009). *Common terminology criteria for adverse events* [v.4.02]. Retrieved August 20, 2009, from http://evs.nci.nih.gov/ftp1/CTCAE/CTCAE_4.02_2009-09-15_QuickReference_8.5x11.pdf

National Comprehensive Cancer Network. (2009). *NCCN Clinical Practice Guidelines in Oncology™: Cancer-related fatigue* [v.1.2009]. Retrieved November 23, 2009, from http://www.nccn.org/professionals/physician_gls/PDF/fatigue.pdf

Natural Medicines Comprehensive Database. (n.d.). *Fatigue.* Retrieved August 20, 2009, from http://www.naturaldatabase.com

Natural Standard Database. (n.d.). *Malaise and related conditions.* Retrieved August 20, 2009, from http://www.naturalstandard.com

Hormonal Changes and Hot Flashes

Introduction

Menopause is defined as the cessation of menstrual cycles for 12 consecutive months. Symptom severity varies. An early sign is irregular menses. As estrogen levels decline, insomnia, headaches, joint pain, vaginal dryness, tiredness, anxiety, irritability, mood swings, depression, loss of libido and memory, and concentration difficulties can occur with a range of severity and intensity. Sweats and hot flashes are common in cancer survivors. The broad-based treatment options include hormonal agents, nonhormonal pharmacotherapies, and diverse integrative medicine modalities.

Sweats are considered to be part of the hot flash complex and exemplify the vasomotor instability seen in menopause. Hot flashes occur in patients with breast cancer (Carpenter et al., 1998). Causes of menopause in the patient with cancer may be surgery, cytotoxic chemotherapy, radiation, or androgen treatment. Causes of "male menopause" include orchiectomy or use of gonadotropin-releasing hormone or estrogen. Tamoxifen, aromatase inhibitors, opioids, tricyclic antidepressants, and steroids can also cause sweats.

Toxicity grading for this symptom according to the CTCAE (NCI CTEP, 2009) can be added to the clinical assessment and reported in the medical record (see Table 17). The following CAM therapies have been evaluated for safety and efficacy.

Table 17. Common Terminology Criteria for Adverse Events: Hot Flashes (Vascular Disorders)

Adverse Event	Grade				
	1	2	3	4	5
Hot flashes	Mild symptoms; intervention not indicated	Moderate symptoms; limiting instrumental ADL	Severe symptoms; limiting self-care ADL	–	–

ADL—activities of daily living

Note. From *Common Terminology Criteria for Adverse Events* [v.4.02] (p. 77), by National Cancer Institute Cancer Therapy Evaluation Program, 2009. Retrieved November 23, 2009, from http://evs.nci.nih.gov/ftp1/CTCAE/CTCAE_4.02_2009-09-15_QuickReference_8.5x11.pdf.

Evidence for Practice

Evidence	Natural Standard	Natural Medicines Comprehensive Database	Physician Data Query
Strong Scientific Evidence	• None reported	• None reported	• Time-limited hormone replacement therapy except in women with breast cancer

Good to Moderate Scientific Evidence	• Menopausal symptoms
	  – Sage
	  – Soy
	• Hot flashes in men
	  – None reported
		• Possibly effective
		  – Flaxseed
		  – Soy (foods)
		• Possibly safe
		  – Black cohosh
		  – Soy (extracts)
			• Alpha adrenergic agonists
			• Androgens
			• Beta-blockers
			• Gabapentin
			• Nonestrogenic, pharmacologic treatment interventions
			• Progestational agents
			• Relaxation therapy
			• Selective serotonin reuptake inhibitors
			• Vitamin E

Weak, Negative, or Conflicting Scientific Evidence	• Acupuncture (hot flashes in men)
	• Alfalfa
	• Androstenediol (testosterone imbalances)
	• Anise for andropause
	• Anise for female menopausal symptoms
	• Ayurveda
	• Black cohosh (hot flashes in men and women)
	• Black currant
	• Black haw
	• Black horehound
	• Borage seed oil
	• Boron
	• Bowen therapy
	• Bupleurum
	• Carrot
	• Chasteberry
		• Insufficient evidence
		  – Alfalfa
		  – Chasteberry
		  – Ginkgo biloba
		  – Hops
		  – Kudzu
		  – Licorice
		  – St. John's wort
		  – Valerian
		  – Vitamin E
		• Possibly ineffective
		  – DHEA
		  – Dong quai
		  – Evening primrose oil
		  – Red clover
		  – Wild yam
			• For women
			  – Black cohosh
			  – Soy
			  – Venlafaxine
			• For men
			  – Estrogens
			  – Gabapentin
			  – Progesterone
			  – Selective serotonin reuptake inhibitors

(Continued on next page)

Evidence	Natural Standard	Natural Medicines Comprehensive Database	Physician Data Query
Weak, Negative, or Conflicting Scientific Evidence (cont.)	• Cleavers • Dandelion • Deer velvet • Devil's claw • DHEA • Dong quai • Echinacea • Evening primrose oil • Fenugreek • Flaxseed • Flaxseed oil • Gamma-linolenic acid • Gamma oryzanol • Garlic • Ginseng • Glyconutrients • Gotu kola • Green tea • Hops • 5-HTP • Hypnotherapy, hypnosis • Ignatia • Kava • Kundalini yoga • Kudzu • Lady's mantle • Lavender • Licorice • Macrobiotic diet • Magnet therapy • Meditation • Milk thistle • Neem (antiestrogen effect) • Nux vomica • Omega-3 fatty acids, fish oil, alpha-linolenic acid • Peony • Polarity therapy • Pomegranate • Prayer, distant healing • Red clover • Reflexology • Relaxation therapy • Resveratrol • Rhodiola		

(Continued on next page)

Evidence	Natural Standard	Natural Medicines Comprehensive Database	Physician Data Query
Weak, Negative, or Conflicting Scientific Evidence (cont.)	• Saw palmetto (hormone imbalances in men and women) • Schissandra • Skullcap • Selenium • Traditional Chinese medicine • Tribulus • Valerian • Vitamin B_6 • Vitamin E • Wild yam • Witch hazel • Tallow dock • Zinc		

Examples of Ongoing Science

Cochrane Collaboration Systematic Reviews

• None at this time

Cochrane Collaboration Protocols

• None at this time
   Complete systematic review and protocol information may be accessed at www.cochrane.org/index.htm.

Examples of Clinical Trials

• Breathe for Hot Flashes (No phase specified. Supportive care. Sponsors: NCI, Other. Protocol IDs: 0803-13, Grant No.: 1R01 CA132927-01, NCT00819182. Active.)
• Soy Derivatives for Control of Hot Flashes in Men on Androgen Deprivation Therapy (Phase II. Supportive care. Sponsor: Other. Protocol IDs: 9639, NCT00594620. Active.)
   Complete clinical trial information may be accessed at http://cancer.gov/clinicaltrials.

Special Considerations

Pediatrics

Little is known about hot flashes in children with cancer. Hormone changes are relative to the cancer site treated. Survivorship issues and research continue with long-term survivors.

Older Adults

Information regarding hormone therapy in men older than 70 years is limited. Side effects that can affect quality of life include hot flashes (O'Rourke, 2006).

Summary

Despite advances in traditional and CAM therapies that may decrease the well-documented discomfort and quality-of-life impact associated with hormone changes and hot flashes, much remains to be learned regarding safe and effective interventions in long-term survivors of childhood cancers and older adults, including older men with prostate cancer. The impact of soy and phytonutrients and other CAM therapies remains controversial.

References

Carpenter, J.S., Andrykowski, M.A., Cordova, M., Cunningham, L., Studts, J., McGrath, P., et al. (1998). Hot flashes in postmenopausal women treated for breast carcinoma: Prevalence, severity, correlates, management, and relation to quality of life. *Cancer, 82*(9), 1682–1691.

National Cancer Institute. (2009). *Fever, sweats, and hot flashes (PDQ®)* [Health professional version]. Retrieved August 20, 2009, from http://www.cancer.gov/cancertopics/pdq/supportive care

National Cancer Institute Cancer Therapy Evaluation Program. (2009). *Common terminology criteria for adverse events* [v.4.02]. Retrieved August 20, 2009, from http://evs.nci.nih.gov/ftp1/ CTCAE/CTCAE_4.02_2009-09-15_QuickReference_8.5x11.pdf

Natural Medicines Comprehensive Databa[se. (n.d.). Retrieved August 20, 2009, from http:// naturaldatabase.therapeuticresearch.com/nd/Search.aspx?cs=&s=ND&pt=9&Product=Hot +flashes&btnSearch.x=17&btnSearch.y=9

Natural Standard Database. (n.d.). Retrieved August 20, 2009, from http://www.naturalstandard .com

O'Rourke, M.E. (2006). The older adult with prostate cancer. In D.G. Cope & A.M. Reb (Eds.), *An evidence-based approach to the treatment and care of the older adult with cancer* (pp. 225–249). Pittsburgh, PA: Oncology Nursing Society.

Insomnia (Sleep-Wake Disturbances)

Introduction

Insomnia is a disorder characterized by difficulty falling asleep and/or remaining asleep (NCI, 2009). It is often a symptom of another underlying condition and frequently situational circumstances such as jet lag, shift work, stress, poor sleep habits, or use of stimulants such as caffeine or other drugs. The four typical types are (a) difficulty falling asleep, (b) difficulty maintaining sleep, (c) early morning awakening, and (d) unrefreshing sleep. All types can cause daytime sleepiness and potentially decrease productivity and increase the risk of accidents.

Toxicity grading for this symptom according to the CTCAE (NCI CTEP, 2009) can be added to the clinical evaluation and reported in the medical record. The criteria range from mild disturbances (grade 1) to severe disturbances (grade 3) (see Table 18).

Evidence for Practice

Successful conventional interventions are available to treat insomnia as seen in *Putting Evidence Into Practice: Improving Oncology Patient Outcomes*

Adverse Event	Grade				
	1	2	3	4	5
Insomnia	Mild difficulty falling asleep, staying asleep, or waking up early	Moderate difficulty falling asleep, staying asleep, or waking up early	Severe difficulty falling asleep, staying asleep, or waking up early	–	–

Table 18. Common Terminology Criteria for Adverse Events: Insomnia

Note. From *Common Terminology Criteria for Adverse Events* [v.4.02] (p. 57), by National Cancer Institute Cancer Therapy Evaluation Program, 2009. Retrieved November 23, 2009, from http://evs.nci.nih.gov/ftp1/CTCAE/CTCAE_4.02_2009-09-15_QuickReference_8.5x11.pdf.

(Page, Berger, & Johnson, 2009). Patients who choose to augment conventional approaches have several economical, safe, and effective CAM options.

Evidence	Natural Standard	Natural Medicines Comprehensive Database	Physician Data Query
Strong Scientific Evidence	• Melatonin (for jet lag)	• None at this time	• None at this time
Good to Moderate Scientific Evidence	• Melatonin (for insomnia in older adults) • Music therapy	• Melatonin • Valerian	• None at this time
Weak, Negative, or Conflicting Scientific Evidence	• 5-HTP • Acupressure, shiatsu • Acupuncture • Aromatherapy (lavender) • Chamomile • Guided imagery • Hypnosis • Valerian	• Hops • Indian snakeroot • Kava • L-tryptophan	• The use of melatonin to treat insomnia in patients with cancer is under evaluation.

Examples of Ongoing Science

Cochrane Collaboration Systematic Reviews

• Acupuncture for Insomnia (Cheuk, Yeung, Chung, & Wong, 2007)

Cochrane Collaboration Protocols

• None at this time
  Complete systematic review and protocol information may be accessed at www.cochrane.org/index.htm.

Examples of Clinical Trials

• Measuring Sleep Disturbance Among Cancer Patients (No phase specified. Supportive care. Sponsor: M.D. Anderson Cancer Center. Protocol IDs: 2004-0598, NCT00505544. Active.)
• Study of Insomnia in Patients Undergoing Chemoradiotherapy for Head and Neck Cancer (No phase specified. Sponsors: Vanderbilt-Ingram Can-

cer Center, NCI. Protocol IDs: VU-VICC-SUPP-0742, NCT00616590. Suspended.)

Complete clinical trial information may be accessed at http://cancer.gov/clinicaltrials.

Special Considerations

Pediatrics

Sleep disorders in children and teens are largely underdiagnosed. Children who snore, have problems falling asleep, are difficult to wake in the morning, or fall asleep in school should be further evaluated for sleep disorders. Considering that sleep problems in children can adversely affect their learning, growth, and development, HCPs should receive education and support in the diagnosis and treatment of sleep disorders (Pradesh, 2009).

Older Adults

Older adults often have problems sleeping, including difficulty falling asleep, waking up during the night, and waking up very early in the morning. At least half of older adults use over-the-counter or prescription medications to help them sleep (American Geriatrics Society Foundation for Health in Aging, 2009). Nonpharmacologic treatment of sleep disorders is the preferred initial management. As long as older adults feel refreshed when they awaken, they are likely getting enough sleep. Providing a regular schedule of meals, discouraging daytime naps, and encouraging physical activity may improve sleep (American Geriatrics Society Foundation for Health in Aging).

Summary

Patients undergoing treatment for cancer often report insomnia. Conventional interventions ameliorating this symptom are safe and effective. Numerous self-help interventions are available to alleviate the severity and duration of insomnia in patients undergoing therapy. CAM interventions are emerging with a supportive scientific basis for incorporation into practice.

References

American Geriatrics Society Foundation for Health in Aging. (2009). *Insomnia*. Retrieved August 20, 2009, from http://www.healthinaging.org/agingintheknow/chapters/ch_31.asp

Cheuk, D.K.L., Yeung, J., Chung, K., & Wong, V. (2007). Acupuncture for insomnia. *Cochrane Database of Systematic Reviews* 2007, Issue 3. Art. No.: CD005472. DOI: 10.1002/14651858. CD005472.pub2.

National Cancer Institute. (2009). *Sleep disorders (PDQ®)* [Health professional version]. Retrieved August 20, 2009, from http://www.cancer.gov/cancertopics/pdq/supportivecare/sleep disorders/healthprofessional/allpages

National Cancer Institute Cancer Therapy Evaluation Program. (2009). *Common terminology criteria for adverse events* [v.4.02]. Retrieved August 20, 2009, from http://evs.nci.nih.gov/ftp1/CTCAE/CTCAE_4.02_2009-09-15_QuickReference_8.5x11.pdf

Natural Medicines Comprehensive Database. (n.d.). *Natural product effectiveness checker: Insomnia.* Retrieved August 20, 2009, from http://naturaldatabase.therapeuticresearch.com

Natural Standard Database. (n.d.). *Insomnia.* Retrieved August 20, 2009, from http://www.natural standard.com

Page, M.S., Berger, A.M., & Johnson, L.B. (2009). ONS PEP resource: Sleep-wake disturbances. In L.H. Eaton & J.M. Tipton (Eds.). *Putting evidence into practice: Improving oncology patient outcomes* (pp. 291–297). Pittsburgh, PA: Oncology Nursing Society.

Pradesh, A. (2009). *Sleep disorders in children are largely under-diagnosed.* Retrieved September 8, 2009, from http://www.andhranews.net/Health/2009/June/8-Sleep-disorders-10206.asp

Mucositis

Introduction

Mucositis is a disorder characterized by inflammation of the oral mucosa (NCI, 2009). Mucositis produces not only discomfort and pain but also can lead to poor nutrition, delays in drug administration, and increased hospital stays and costs. Mucositis first appears and often is most severe on the mucosa of the soft palate, tonsillar pillars, buccal mucosa, lateral border of the tongue, and pharyngeal walls. After chemotherapy, GI mucositis is most prominent in the small intestine but also occurs in the esophagus, stomach, and large intestine. Radiation esophagitis and radiation proctitis are manifestations of GI mucositis (Sonis et al., 2004).

Multiple grading systems for mucositis exist with varying levels of ranking both oral and GI mucositis. Toxicity grading for this symptom according to the CTCAE (NCI CTEP, 2009) can be added to the clinical evaluation and reported in the medical record. The criteria range from asymptomatic (grade 1) to life-threatening consequences (grade 4) to death (grade 5) (see Table 19).

Table 19. Common Terminology Criteria for Adverse Events: Mucositis					
Adverse Event	**Grade**				
	1	**2**	**3**	**4**	**5**
Mucositis oral	Asymptomatic or mild symptoms; intervention not indicated	Moderate pain; not interfering with oral intake; modified diet indicated	Severe pain; interfering with oral intake	Life-threatening consequences; urgent intervention indicated	Death

Note. From *Common Terminology Criteria for Adverse Events* [v.4.02] (p. 18), by National Cancer Institute Cancer Therapy Evaluation Program, 2009. Retrieved November 23, 2009, from http://evs.nci.nih.gov/ftp1/CTCAE/CTCAE_4.02_2009-09-15_QuickReference_8.5x11.pdf.

Evidence for Practice

Conventional interventions to treat mucositis are aimed at symptom relief and preventing further tissue damage as seen in *Putting Evidence Into Practice: Improving Oncology Patient Outcomes* (Harris, Eilers, Cashavelly, Maxwell, & Harriman, 2009). Patients who choose to augment conventional approaches have several economical, safe, and effective CAM therapy options available.

Evidence	Natural Standard	Natural Medicines Comprehensive Database	Physician Data Query
Strong Scientific Evidence	• None at this time	• None at this time	• None at this time
Good to Moderate Scientific Evidence	• Iodine	• Hyaluronic acid	• None at this time
Weak, Negative, or Conflicting Scientific Evidence	• Chamomile	• German chamomile • Glutamine • Iodine • Kaolin	• Allopurinol mouthwash • Cryotherapy (with fluorouracil chemotherapy)

Examples of Ongoing Science

Cochrane Collaboration Systematic Reviews

- Interventions for Preventing Oral Mucositis for Patients With Cancer Receiving Treatment (Worthington, Clarkson, & Eden, 2007)

Cochrane Collaboration Protocols

- Glutamine Supplementation in Enteral or Parenteral Nutrition for the Incidence of Mucositis in Colorectal Cancer (Pinto de Lemos, Lemos, Atallah, & Soares, 2004)

  Complete systematic review and protocol information may be accessed at www.cochrane.org/index.htm.

Examples of Clinical Trials

- A Trial of Homeopathic Medication TRAUMEEL S for the Treatment of Radiation-Induced Mucositis (Phase I. Supportive care. Sponsor: University of Oklahoma. Protocol IDs: TRAUMEEL_S_Krempl, NCT00584597. Active.)

- Curcumin for Prevention of Oral Mucositis in Children Receiving Doxorubicin-Based Chemotherapy (Phase III. Supportive care treatment. Sponsor: Hadassah Medical Organization. Protocol IDs: Curcumin-HMO-CTIL, NCT00475683. Active.)

  Complete clinical trial information may be accessed at http://cancer.gov/clinicaltrials.

Special Considerations

Pediatrics

In children receiving chemotherapy, the incidence of oral mucositis is reported to be 52%–80% (Cheng & Chang, 2003). Oral infections and tooth decay during chemotherapy can be prevented with diligent oral care, but this is challenging in this age group. Novel therapies for the relief of mucositis-related complications are needed in this population (Ped-Onc Resource Center, 2005).

Older Adults

Age-related changes such as decreased salivary flow, increased gingivitis and decreased mucosal keratinization may contribute to the known increased risk of severe oral and GI mucositis (Balducci & Corcoran, 2000).

Summary

Mucositis commonly occurs in patients who are treated with cytotoxic therapy or radiation therapy. Well-designed, controlled, and standardized studies are necessary to validate effectiveness of available as well as newly developed interventions for mucositis. Conventional interventions ameliorating this symptom are safe and effective. CAM interventions are emerging with a supportive scientific basis for incorporation into practice.

References

Balducci, L., & Corcoran, M.B. (2000). Antineoplastic chemotherapy of the older cancer patient. *Hematology/Oncology Clinics of North America, 14*(1), 193–212.

Cheng, K.K., & Chang, A.M. (2003). Palliation of oral mucositis symptoms in pediatric patients treated with cancer chemotherapy. *Cancer Nursing, 26*(6), 476–484.

Harris, D.J., Eilers, J.G., Cashavelly, B.J., Maxwell, C.L., & Harriman, A. (2009). ONS PEP resource: Mucositis. In L.H. Eaton & J.M. Tipton (Eds.), *Putting evidence into practice: Improving oncology patient outcomes* (pp. 201–213). Pittsburgh, PA: Oncology Nursing Society.

National Cancer Institute. (2009). *Oral complications of chemotherapy and head/neck radiation (PDQ®): Oral mucositis* [Health professional version]. Retrieved August 20, 2009, from http://www.cancer.gov/cancertopics/pdq/supportivecare/oralcomplications/HealthProfessional/page6

National Cancer Institute Cancer Therapy Evaluation Program. (2009). *Common terminology criteria for adverse events* [v.4.02]. Retrieved August 20, 2009, from http://evs.nci.nih.gov/ftp1/CTCAE/CTCAE_4.02_2009-09-15_QuickReference_8.5x11.pdf

Natural Medicines Comprehensive Database. (n.d.). *Natural product effectiveness checker: Mucositis.* Retrieved August 20, 2009, from http://naturaldatabase.therapeuticresearch.com/nd/Search.aspx?cs=CE_NODEACT&s=ND&pt=9&Product=mucositis

Natural Standard Database. (n.d.). *Conditions monograph: Mucositis.* Retrieved August 20, 2009, from http://www.naturalstandard.com

Ped-Onc Resource Center. (2005, August). *Mouth and teeth: Care and problems.* Retrieved September 8, 2009, from http://www.acor.org/ped-onc/treatment/mouthcare.html

Pinto de Lemos, H., Lemos, A.L.A., Atallah, Á.N., & Soares, B. (2004). Glutamine supplementation in enteral or parenteral nutrition for the incidence of mucositis in colorectal cancer (Protocol). *Cochrane Database of Systematic Reviews* 2004, Issue 1. Art. No.: CD004650. DOI: 10.1002/14651858.CD004650.

Sonis, S.T., Elting, L.S., Keefe, D., Peterson, D.E., Schubert, M., Hauer-Jensen, M., et al. (2004). Perspectives on cancer therapy-induced mucosal injury: pathogenesis, measurement, epidemiology, and consequences for patients. *Cancer, 100*(Suppl. 9), 1995–2025.

Worthington, H.V., Clarkson, J.E., & Eden, T.O.B. (2007). Interventions for preventing oral mucositis for patients with cancer receiving treatment. *Cochrane Database of Systematic Reviews* 2007, Issue 4. Art. No.: CD000978. DOI: 10.1002/14651858.CD000978.pub3.

Myelosuppression

Introduction

Myelosuppression is a reduction in bone marrow function resulting in a reduced production of red blood cells, white blood cells (WBCs), and platelets into the peripheral circulation and includes anemia, neutropenia, and thrombocytopenia. Anemia is a disorder characterized by a reduction in the amount of hemoglobin in 100 ml of blood (NCI CTEP, 2009). Neutropenia is a condition in which the total number of circulatory WBCs is decreased, which may lead to an increased risk of infection. Thrombocytopenia is a condition in which the number of platelets is less than normal, which may cause an increased risk of oozing, bruising, and bleeding. Myelosuppression, considered to be the most common dose-limiting side effect of cancer therapy, can be a complex experience involving fatigue, infection, shortness of breath, body image changes, and overall alterations in quality of life.

Toxicity grading for this symptom according to the CTCAE (NCI CTEP, 2009) can be added to the clinical evaluation and reported in the medical record. The criteria range from asymptomatic (grade 1) to life-threatening consequences (grade 4) to death (grade 5) (see Table 20).

Table 20. Common Terminology Criteria for Adverse Events: Blood and Lymphatic System Disorders

Adverse Event	Grade				
	1	2	3	4	5
Anemia	Hemoglobin < LLN–10.0 g/dl; < LLN–6.2 mmol/L; < LLN–100 g/L	Hemoglobin < 10.0–8.0 g/dl; < 6.2–4.9 mmol/L; < 100–80 g/L	Hemoglobin < 8.0–6.5; < 4.9–4.0 mmol/L; < 80–65 g/L; transfusion indicated	Life-threatening consequences; urgent intervention indicated	Death

(Continued on next page)

119

Table 20. Common Terminology Criteria for Adverse Events: Blood and Lymphatic System Disorders *(Continued)*

Adverse Event	Grade				
	1	2	3	4	5
Leuko-cytes (total WBC)	< LLN–3,000/mm³ < LLN–3.0 × 10⁹/L	<3,000–2,000/mm³ < 3.0–2.0 × 10⁹/L	2,000–1,000/mm³ < 2.0–1.0 × 10⁹/L	< 1,000/mm³ < 1.0 × 10⁹/L	Death
Platelets	< LLN–75,000/mm³ < LLN–75.0 × 10⁹/L	< 75,000–50,000/mm³ < 75.0–50.0 × 10⁹/L	< 50,000–20,000/mm³ < 50.0–25.0 × 10⁹/L	< 25,000/mm³ < 25.0 × 10⁹/L	Death

LLN—lower limit of normal; WBC—white blood cells

Note. From *Common Terminology Criteria for Adverse Events* [v.4.02] (p. 3), by National Cancer Institute Cancer Therapy Evaluation Program, 2009. Retrieved November 23, 2009, from http://evs.nci.nih.gov/ftp1/CTCAE/CTCAE_4.02_2009-09-15_QuickReference_8.5x11.pdf.

Evidence for Practice

Successful conventional interventions are available to treat myelosuppression.

Evidence	Natural Standard	Natural Medicines Comprehensive Database	Physician Data Query
Strong Scientific Evidence	• Anemia: folate, iron, liver extract, vitamin B₁₂, vitamin B₆, zinc	• Anemia of chronic disease: iron • Iron-deficiency anemia: iron • Pernicious anemia: vitamin B₁₂	• None at this time
Good to Moderate Scientific Evidence	• Anemia: iron	• Anemia: vitamin E	• None at this time
Weak, Negative, or Conflicting Scientific Evidence	• Antineoplastics (sickle-cell anemia, thalassemia) • Copper (sideroblastic anemia) • Iron (anemia of chronic disease)	• Anemia: histidine, vitamin A • Leukopenia: echinacea	• None at this time

(Continued on next page)

Evidence	Natural Standard	Natural Medicines Comprehensive Database	Physician Data Query
Weak, Negative, or Conflicting Scientific Evidence (cont.)	• L-carnitine (sickle-cell anemia) • Prayer (sickle-cell anemia) • Taurine (iron-deficiency anemia) • Vitamin A (iron-deficiency anemia) • Vitamin B_{12} (iron-deficiency anemia)		

Examples of Ongoing Science

Cochrane Collaboration Systematic Reviews

• None at this time

Cochrane Collaboration Protocols

• None at this time

Complete systematic review and protocol information may be accessed at www.cochrane.org/index.htm.

Examples of Clinical Trials

• None at this time

Complete clinical trial information may be accessed at http://cancer.gov/clinicaltrials.

Special Considerations

Pediatrics

The COG Nutrition Committee is furthering the knowledge of nutrition in children with cancer by education and the conduct of clinical trials. COG has developed an algorithm as a guideline for nutritional intervention (Children's Hospital of New York-Presbyterian, 2009).

Older Adults

Anemia is the most common age-related hematologic abnormality in older men and women, and many comprehensive workups fail to identify a cause. Studies have shown that a reduction in hemoglobin is related to lower neutrophil levels and can serve as a marker of decreased overall hematopoietic reserve capacity. Evaluation of anemia when values are less than 10.5 g/dl in an older adult with cancer invariably identifies a pathologic cause; thus, prompt attention is warranted (American Geriatrics Society, 2009).

Anemia may increase the risk for adverse drug reactions, risk of delirium, and complications from cytotoxic chemotherapy (Balducci, 2003).

Thrombocytopenia is a common cause of bleeding problems in older adults and can present as unexplained bruises, nosebleeds, or GI losses. Bleeding can occur when the platelet count drops to 20,000/microliter or less. Immune thrombocytopenia is usually a secondary presentation in older adults, so the initial approach is to identify and treat the primary cause (American Geriatrics Society, 2009).

Summary

Myelosuppression can be a complex experience involving fatigue, infection, shortness of breath, body image changes, and overall alterations in quality of life. Conventional interventions ameliorating this symptom are safe and effective. CAM interventions are emerging with a supportive scientific basis for incorporation into practice.

References

American Geriatrics Society. (2009). *Palliative care*. Retrieved December 22, 2009, from http://www.healthinaging.org/agingintheknow/oldfiles/Ch_16_Pallativecare_hospice.htm

Balducci, L. (2003). Myelosuppression and its consequences in elderly patients with cancer. *Oncology, 17*(Suppl. 11), 27–32.

Children's Hospital of New York-Presbyterian. (2009). *Integrative Therapies Program for Children With Cancer, 2009.* Retrieved August 20, 2009, from http://integrativetherapies.columbia.edu

National Cancer Institute Cancer Therapy Evaluation Program. (2009). *Common terminology criteria for adverse events* [v.4.02]. Retrieved August 20, 2009, from http://evs.nci.nih.gov/ftp1/CTCAE/CTCAE_4.02_2009-09-15_QuickReference_8.5x11.pdf

Natural Medicines Comprehensive Database. (n.d.). *Natural product effectiveness checker: Myelosuppression*. Retrieved August 20, 2009, from http://www.naturaldatabase.com

Natural Standard Database. (n.d.). *Aplastic anemia and related conditions*. Retrieved August 20, 2009, from http://www.naturalstandard.com

Nausea and Vomiting

Introduction

Nausea is a disorder characterized by a queasy sensation and the urge to vomit (NCI, 2009). *Vomiting* is a disorder characterized by the reflexive act of ejecting the contents of the stomach through the mouth (NCI). Nausea is considered to be a more frequent and perhaps more significant problem because it is under-assessed and more poorly controlled than vomiting (Wickham, 2004).

Toxicity grading for this symptom according to the CTCAE (NCI CTEP, 2009) can be added to the clinical evaluation and reported in the medical record. The CTCAE criteria for nausea range from loss of appetite without alteration in eating habits (grade 1) to inadequate intake requiring nutritional intervention or hospitalization (grade 3). For vomiting, the criteria range from few episodes (grade 1) to life-threatening consequences (grade 4) to death (grade 5) (see Table 21).

Table 21. Common Terminology Criteria for Adverse Events: Gastrointestinal Disorders

Adverse Event	Grade				
	1	2	3	4	5
Nausea	Loss of appetite without alteration in eating habits	Oral intake decreased without significant weight loss, dehydration, or malnutrition	Inadequate oral caloric or fluid intake; tube feeding, TPN, or hospitalization indicated	–	–
Vomiting	1–2 episodes (separated by 5 minutes) in 24 hours	3–5 episodes (separated by 5 minutes) in 24 hours	≥ 6 episodes (separated by 5 minutes) in 24 hours; tube feeding, TPN, or hospitalization indicated	Life-threatening consequences; urgent intervention indicated	Death

TPN—total parenteral nutrition

Note. From *Common Terminology Criteria for Adverse Events* [v.4.02] (pp. 18, 21), by National Cancer Institute Cancer Therapy Evaluation Program, 2009. Retrieved November 23, 2009, from http://evs.nci.nih.gov/ftp1/CTCAE/CTCAE_4.02_2009-09-15_QuickReference_8.5x11.pdf.

Evidence for Practice

Successful conventional interventions are available to treat nausea and vomiting as seen in *Putting Evidence Into Practice: Improving Oncology Patient Outcomes* (Friend et al., 2009). Patients who choose to augment conventional approaches have several economical, safe, and effective CAM nutritional therapy options available.

Evidence	Natural Standard	Natural Medicines Comprehensive Database	Physician Data Query
Strong Scientific Evidence	• Acupressure, shiatsu	• None at this time	• None at this time
Good to Moderate Scientific Evidence	• Acupuncture • Acustimulation • Ginger • Music therapy	• Acupuncture for chemotherapy-induced nausea and vomiting (CINV) • Ginger for postoperative nausea and vomiting	• Electroacupuncture for acute vomiting • Guided imagery and hypnosis for anticipatory nausea and vomiting
Weak, Negative, or Conflicting Scientific Evidence	• Hypnosis • Peppermint • Transdermal electrical nerve stimulation	• Acupressure for CINV	• Acupressure for acute nausea • Behavioral therapy • Guided imagery • Hypnosis • Relaxation techniques

Examples of Ongoing Science

Cochrane Collaboration Systematic Reviews

• Acupuncture-Point Stimulation for Chemotherapy-Induced Nausea or Vomiting (Ezzo et al., 2006)

Cochrane Collaboration Protocols

• Aromatherapy for Treatment of Postoperative Nausea and Vomiting (Hines, Steels, Chang, & Gilshenan, 2009)

Complete systematic review and protocol information may be accessed at www.cochrane.org/index.htm.

Examples of Clinical Trials

- Electroacupuncture for Treating Delayed Nausea and Vomiting in Patients Receiving Chemotherapy for Newly Diagnosed Childhood Sarcoma, Neuroblastoma, Nasopharyngeal Carcinoma, Germ Cell Tumors, or Hodgkin Lymphoma (No phase specified. Supportive care. Sponsors: National Center for Complementary and Alternative Medicine, NCI. Protocol IDs: NCCAM-02-AT-0172, NCI-02-AT-0172, COG-ACCL04C2, ACCL04C2, NCT00040911. Active.)
- Phase II Randomized Study of Acupuncture in Reducing Postoperative Ileus in Patients Who Have Undergone Surgery for Colorectal Cancer (Phase II. Supportive Care. Sponsors: Memorial Sloan-Kettering Cancer Center, NCI. Protocol IDs: MSKCC-06145, NCT00425412. Active.)

Complete clinical trial information may be accessed at http://cancer.gov/clinicaltrials.

Special Considerations

Pediatrics

The COG Nutrition Committee is furthering the knowledge of nutrition in children with cancer by education and the conduct of clinical trials. COG has developed an algorithm as a guideline for nutritional intervention (Children's Hospital of New York-Presbyterian, 2009).

Older Adults

Evaluation and prompt intervention of nausea and vomiting are necessary if related to chemotherapy. If the patient is not seriously ill or dehydrated, assessment on an outpatient basis for spontaneous, non–treatment-related nausea or vomiting can possibly be delayed for 24–48 hours. Earlier intervention or hospitalization may be required for patients who are seriously ill (American Geriatrics Society, 2009).

Summary

Nausea and vomiting commonly occur in patients with cancer. Conventional interventions ameliorating these symptoms are safe and effective. CAM interventions are emerging with a supportive scientific basis for incorporation into practice.

References

American Geriatrics Society. (2009). *Palliative care*. Retrieved August 20, 2009, from http://www.americangeriatrics.org

Children's Hospital of New York-Presbyterian. (2009). *The Integrative Therapies Program for Children With Cancer, 2009.* Retrieved August 20, 2009, from http://integrativetherapies.columbia.edu

Ezzo, J., Richardson, M.A., Vickers, A., Allen, C., Dibble, S., Issell, B.F., et al. (2006). Acupuncture-point stimulation for chemotherapy-induced nausea or vomiting. *Cochrane Database of Systematic Reviews* 2006, Issue 2. Art. No.: CD002285. DOI: 10.1002/14651858.CD002285.pub2.

Friend, P.J., Johnston, M.P., Tipton, J.M., McDaniel, R.W., Barbour, L.A., Starr, P., et al. (2009). ONS PEP resource: Chemotherapy-induced nausea and vomiting. In L.H. Eaton & J.M. Tipton (Eds.), *Putting evidence into practice: Improving oncology patient outcomes* (pp. 71–83). Pittsburgh, PA: Oncology Nursing Society.

Hines, S., Steels, E., Chang, A., & Gilshenan, K. (2009). Aromatherapy for treatment of postoperative nausea and vomiting (Protocol). *Cochrane Database of Systematic Reviews* 2009, Issue 1. Art. No.: CD007598. DOI: 10.1002/14651858.CD007598.

National Cancer Institute. (2009). *Nausea and Vomiting (PDQ®).* Retrieved August 20, 2009, from http://www.cancer.gov/cancertopics/pdq/supportivecare/nausea/patient/allpages

National Cancer Institute Cancer Therapy Evaluation Program. (2009). *Common terminology criteria for adverse events* [v.4.02]. Retrieved August 20, 2009, from http://evs.nci.nih.gov/ftp1/CTCAE/CTCAE_4.02_2009-09-15_QuickReference_8.5x11.pdf

Natural Medicines Comprehensive Database. (n.d.). *Natural product effectiveness checker: Nausea.* Retrieved August 20, 2009, from http://www.naturaldatabase.com

Natural Standard Database. (n.d.). *Conditions monograph: Nausea and vomiting.* Retrieved August 20, 2009, from http://www.naturalstandard.com

Wickham, R. (2004). Nausea and vomiting. In C.H. Yarbro, M.H. Frogge, & M. Goodman (Eds.), *Cancer symptom management* (3rd ed., pp. 187–214). Sudbury, MA: Jones and Bartlett.

Pain

Introduction

Pain is an unpleasant sensory and sometimes emotional feeling associated with actual or potential tissue damage. Pain is considered the most feared of all symptoms associated with cancer.

Unrelieved pain can affect all facets of an individual's life. Studies have revealed that multiple other symptoms are associated with cancer pain, such as fatigue, anxiety, and depression. Pain contributes to suffering and has an overall negative effect on quality of life.

Cancer-related causes of pain include the presence of the tumor (metastases), a result of therapy (diagnostic and treatment procedures), and prior or current painful conditions (e.g., arthritis). Types of pain include acute versus chronic; neuropathic versus nociceptive; and somatic, visceral, or psychogenic. Known barriers to therapeutic pain management include misconceptions, misinformation, and mismanagement involving HCPs, healthcare systems, and the public, patients, and families.

Toxicity grading for this symptom according to the CTCAE (NCI CTEP, 2009) can be added to the clinical evaluation and reported in the medical record. The criteria range from mild pain that does not interfere with function (grade 1) to disabling (grade 4). Although pain can occur anywhere in the body, the criteria remain unchanged regardless of the location (see Table 22).

Table 22. Common Terminology Criteria for Adverse Events: Pain					
Adverse Event	**Grade**				
	1	**2**	**3**	**4**	**5**
Pain	Mild pain not interfering with function	Moderation pain; pain or analgesics interfering with function, but not interfering with ADL	Severe pain; pain or analgesics severely interfering with ADL	Disabling	–

ADL—activities of daily living

Note. From *Common Terminology Criteria for Adverse Events* [v.4.02] (p. 23), by National Cancer Institute Cancer Therapy Evaluation Program, 2009. Retrieved November 23, 2009, from http://evs.nci.nih.gov/ftp1/CTCAE/CTCAE_4.02_2009-09-15_QuickReference_8.5x11.pdf.

Evidence for Practice

The use of opioids, nonopioids, and coanalgesics is considered to provide effective management of acute and persistent, nociceptive and neuropathic pain resulting from cancer and the treatment of cancer (American Pain Society, 2005; National Comprehensive Cancer Network, 2009). Patients who choose to augment conventional approaches have limited economical, evidence-based CAM therapy options.

Evidence	Natural Standard	Natural Medicines Comprehensive Database	Physician Data Query
Strong Scientific Evidence	• None reported for cancer pain	• None reported	• Massage (short-term benefits)
Good to Moderate Scientific Evidence	• Cancer pain—none specifically reported • General pain – Guided imagery – Hypnotherapy, hypnosis – Music therapy – Physical therapy – Therapeutic touch • Inflammation—bromelain and comfrey (either separately or in conjunction with each other)	• Camphor (general pain, likely effective) • Capsicum (pain, likely effective) • Magnesium (cancer-associated neuropathic pain) • Reflexology (cancer-associated pain)	• Cognitive behavioral interventions—decrease symptom burden • Relaxation • Imagery • Hypnosis • Cognitive distraction and reframing
Weak, Negative, or Conflicting Scientific Evidence	• Acupuncture (pain, chronic pain) • Acupressure, shiatsu (postoperative pain) • Acustimulation (pain) • Alpha-lipoic acid (burning mouth syndrome) • Arginine (dental pain) • Arnica (postoperative pain) • Bach flower remedies (pain) • Bowen therapy (pain) • Cat's claw (inflammation) • Chiropractic (shoulder, pelvic, and thoracic spine pain)	• Acupuncture (cancer-associated pain) • Adenosine (neuropathic pain) • Qigong (pain) • Reiki (cancer-associated pain) • Therapeutic touch (breast biopsy pain, neuropathic pain) • Therapeutic touch (cancer-associated pain)	• None specifically reported at this time

(Continued on next page)

Evidence	Natural Standard	Natural Medicines Comprehensive Database	Physician Data Query
Weak, Negative, or Conflicting Scientific Evidence (cont.)	• Color therapy (pain) • Dandelion (inflammation) • *Euphorbia* (oral cavity inflammation) • Healing touch (postoperative and chronic pain) • Licorice (inflammation) • Para-aminobenzoic acid (cancer pain) • Prayer, distant healing (chronic pain) • Qigong (pain, chronic pain) • Reiki (pain) • Reishi mushroom (postherpetic pain) • Relaxation (pain) • Spiritual healing (pain) • Therapeutic touch (phantom limb pain) • Turmeric (inflammation) • White horehound (pain) • Yoga (pain) *Pediatric specific* • Aconite(postoperative pain—infants) • Pet therapy (pain)		

Examples of Ongoing Science

Cochrane Collaboration Systematic Reviews

• Music for Pain Relief (Cepeda, Carr, Lau, & Alvarez, 2006)
  – Authors concluded that listening to music reduced pain intensity and opioid requirements.
  – The magnitude of these benefits was small, and implications for clinical practice remain unclear.
• Vitamin D for the Treatment of Painful Conditions in Adults (Straube, Derry, Moore, & McQuay, 2010)

Cochrane Collaboration Protocols

• Acupuncture for Cancer Pain in Adults (Paley, Johnson, Tashani, & Bagnall, 2009)

Complete systematic review and protocol information may be accessed at www.cochrane.org/index.htm.

Examples of Clinical Trials

- Acupuncture in Treating Mucositis-Related Pain Caused by Chemotherapy in Patients Undergoing Hematopoietic Stem Cell Transplantation (No phase specified. Sponsor: NCI. Protocol IDs: NCI-03-0-125, NCT00060021. Closed.)
- Animal-Assisted Therapy and Recreation Therapy in Relieving Distress in Cancer Patients Undergoing Treatment for Pain (No phase specified. Sponsor: NCI. Protocol IDs: NCT00103688, 05-CC-0093. Active.)

Complete clinical trial information may be accessed at http://cancer.gov/clinicaltrials.

Special Considerations

Pediatrics

Despite broad popular interest in complementary and alternative therapies, few children are offered access to these treatments (NCI, 2009). Guided imagery, hypnosis, and biofeedback have been shown to be effective adjuncts to medical therapy (Kemper, Vohra, & Walls, 2010).

Older Adults

Pain assessment may be more complex in older adults because of multiple medical problems, cognitive impairment, underreporting of pain, misconceptions about pain events and pain management, multiple sources of pain, multiple medications with potential interactions, and alterations in pharmacokinetics.

Summary

Pain can be a common occurrence in patients with cancer. Accurate assessment is fundamental when using conventional and CAM therapies. Conventional interventions ameliorating this symptom are safe and effective. CAM interventions are emerging with scientific evidence for incorporation into practice.

References

American Pain Society. (2005). *Guideline for the management of cancer pain in adults and children.* Glenview, IL: Author.

Cepeda, M.S., Carr, D.B., Lau, J., & Alvarez, H. Music for pain relief. *Cochrane Database of Systematic Reviews* 2006, Issue 2. Art. No.: CD004843. DOI: 10.1002/14651858.CD004843.pub2.

Kemper, K.J., Vohra, S., & Walls, R. (2008). American Academy of Pediatrics, Task Force on Complementary, Holistic, and Integrative Medicine. The use of complementary and alternative medicine in pediatrics. *Pediatrics, 122,* 1374–1386.

National Cancer Institute. (2009). *Pain (PDQ®)*. Retrieved January 11, 2009, from http://www.cancer.gov/cancertopics

National Cancer Institute Cancer Therapy Evaluation Program. (2009). *Common terminology criteria for adverse events* [v.4.02]. Retrieved August 20, 2009, from http://evs.nci.nih.gov/ftp1/CTCAE/CTCAE_4.02_2009-09-15_QuickReference_8.5x11.pdf

National Comprehensive Cancer Network. (2009). *NCCN Clinical Practice Guidelines in Oncology™: Adult cancer pain* [v.1.2009]. Retrieved March 26, 2010, from http://www.nccn.org/professionals/physician_gls/PDF/pain.pdf

Natural Medicines Comprehensive Database. (n.d.). *Natural medicines in the clinical management of pain.* Retrieved August 20, 2009, from http://www.naturaldatabase.com

Natural Standard Database. (n.d.). *Pain and related conditions.* Retrieved August 20, 2009, from http://www.naturalstandard.com

Paley, C.A., Johnson, M.I., Tashani, O.A., & Bagnall, A.M. (2009). Acupuncture for cancer pain in adults (Protocol). *Cochrane Database of Systematic Reviews* 2009, Issue 2. Art. No.: CD007753. DOI: 10.1002/14651858.CD007753.

Straube, S., Derry, S., Moore, R.A., & McQuay, H.J. (2010). Vitamin D for the treatment of chronic painful conditions in adults. *Cochrane Database of Systematic Reviews* 2010, Issue 1. Art. No.: CD007771. DOI: 10.1002/14651858.CD007771.pub2.

Sexuality Alterations

Introduction

Sexuality is integral to each person, involving every aspect of the individual and his or her life (Krebs, 2010; Tierney, 2008). In those with cancer, sexual capacity may be affected by a complex set of factors, including cancer and its treatment, comorbidities, and psychosocial issues. Alterations in sexual function include problems with erection and ejaculation in men; dyspareunia, vaginismus, altered vaginal lubrication, and orgasm difficulties in women; and decreased libido and inability to have intercourse in both men and women. All physiologic problems affecting sexuality can be exacerbated by perceived alterations in sexual identity and body image, loss of self-esteem, fears of being abandoned, and concerns about self (Krebs, 2006, 2008).

Multiple sexual assessment and intervention strategies exist, including the PLISSIT (permission, limited information, specific suggestions, intensive therapy) (Annon, 1974), Ex-PLISSIT (extended PLISSIT) (Davis & Taylor, 2006), and BETTER (bringing up the topic, explaining that sexuality is part of quality of life, telling patients that resources will be found to address their concerns, timing the intervention, educating patients about sexual side effects of treatment, and recording) models (Mick, Hughes, & Cohen, 2004). These or similar models should be used to evaluate all patients diagnosed with cancer.

Toxicity grading for sexuality alterations according to the CTCAE (NCI CTEP, 2009) can be added to the clinical assessment and reported in the medical record. Multiple adverse events for aspects of sexual dysfunction include ejaculation disorder, erectile dysfunction (ED), dyspareunia, vaginal discharge, vaginal dryness, vaginismus, anorgasmia, delayed orgasm, and decreased libido. Criteria vary by event and generally range from requiring no to minimal intervention or having no effect on the relationship (grade 1) to affecting the relationship or requiring some form of intervention (grade 2) to severe discomfort (grade 3). Neither life-threatening consequences (grade 4) nor the possibility of death (grade 5) is associated with the sexual dysfunction events (see Table 23).

Table 23. Common Terminology Criteria for Adverse Events: Sexual Dysfunction

Adverse Event	Grade				
	1	2	3	4	5
Men					
Ejaculation disorder	Diminished ejaculation	Anejaculation or retrograde ejaculation	–	–	–
Erectile dysfunction	Decrease in erectile function (frequency or rigidity of erections) but intervention not indicated (e.g., medication or use of mechanical device, penile pump)	Decrease in erectile function (frequency/rigidity of erections), erectile intervention indicated, (e.g., medication or mechanical devices such as penile pump)	Decrease in erectile function (frequency/rigidity of erections) but erectile intervention not helpful (e.g., medication or mechanical devices such as penile pump); placement of a permanent penile prosthesis indicated (not previously present)	–	–
Women					
Anorgasmia	Inability to achieve orgasm not adversely affecting relationship	Inability to achieve orgasm adversely affecting relationship	–	–	–
Delayed orgasm	Delay in achieving orgasm not adversely affecting relationship	Delay in achieving orgasm adversely affecting relationship	–	–	–
Dyspareunia	Mild discomfort or pain associated with vaginal penetration; discomfort relieved with use of vaginal lubricants or estrogen	Moderate discomfort or pain associated with vaginal penetration; discomfort or pain partially relieved with use of vaginal lubricants or estrogen	Severe discomfort or pain associated with vaginal penetration; discomfort or pain unrelieved by vaginal lubricants or estrogen	–	–

(Continued on next page)

Table 23. Common Terminology Criteria for Adverse Events: Sexual Dysfunction *(Continued)*

Adverse Event	Grade				
	1	2	3	4	5
Vaginal discharge	Mild vaginal discharge (greater than baseline for patient)	Moderate to heavy vaginal discharge; use of perineal pad or tampon indicated	–	–	–
Vaginal dryness	Mild vaginal dryness not interfering with sexual function	Moderate vaginal dryness interfering with sexual function or causing frequent discomfort	Severe vaginal dryness resulting in dyspareunia or severe discomfort	–	–
Vaginismus	Mild discomfort or pain associated with vaginal spasm/tightening; no impact upon sexual function or physical examination	Moderate discomfort or pain associated with vaginal spasm/tightening; disruption in sexual function and physical examination	Severe discomfort or pain associated with vaginal spasm/tightening; unable to tolerate vaginal penetration or physical examination	–	–
Men and Women					
Libido decreased	Decrease in sexual interest not adversely affecting relationship	Decrease in sexual interest adversely affecting relationship	–	–	–

Note. From *Common Terminology Criteria for Adverse Events* [v.4.02] (pp. 57, 61–64), by National Cancer Institute Cancer Therapy Evaluation Program, 2009. Retrieved November 23, 2009, from http://evs.nci.nih.gov/ftp1/CTCAE/CTCAE_4.02_2009-09-15_QuickReference_8.5x11.pdf.

Evidence for Practice

Successful conventional interventions are available to treat aspects of sexual dysfunction, including medications, medical devices, and various levels of counseling and lifestyle alterations (Albaugh, Kellogg-Spadt, Krebs, Lewis, & Kramer-Levien, 2009; Katz, 2007; Krebs, 2006, 2008, 2010). Patients who choose to augment conventional approaches have numerous CAM therapy options, some with more scientific evidence of effectiveness than others, with ED being the most studied sexual dysfunction.

Evidence	Natural Standard	Natural Medicines Comprehensive Database	Physician Data Query
Strong Scientific Evidence	• None at this time	• None at this time	• Psychological assessment and treatment (decreased libido)
Good to Moderate Scientific Evidence	• Psychotherapy (sexual dysfunction)	• DHEA, Panax ginseng, L-arginine, melanotan-II, propionyl-L-carnitine, yohimbe (ED) • Yohimbe (sexual dysfunction)	• None at this time
Weak, Negative, or Conflicting Scientific Evidence	• Acupressure • Acupuncture • Arginine • Calcium (vaginal atrophy, thinning) • Clove • Coleus • Cordyceps • Damiana • DHEA • Ephedra • Ginkgo • Ginseng • Horny goat weed • Hypnotherapy • L-carnitine • Maca • Muira puama • Pomegranate • Pycnogenol® (Horphag) • Yoga • Yohimbe bark extract (sexual dysfunction including ED and decreased libido)	• DHEA (sexual arousal disorder) • Ginkgo (sexual dysfunction) • Pycnogenol (ED)	• Brief sexual counseling (ED, dyspareunia) • Support groups (sexual dysfunction)

Examples of Ongoing Science

Cochrane Collaboration Systematic Reviews

• Interventions for Sexual Dysfunction Following Treatments for Cancer (Miles et al., 2007)

- Psychosocial Interventions for Erectile Dysfunction (Melnik, Soares, & Nasello, 2007)
- Interventions for the Physical Aspects of Sexual Dysfunction in Women Following Pelvic Radiotherapy (Denton & Maher, 2003)
- Interventions for Psychosexual Dysfunction in Women Treated for Gynaecological Malignancy (Flynn, Kew, & Kisely, 2009)

Cochrane Collaboration Protocols

- Acupuncture for the Treatment of Erectile Dysfunction (Liu, Fei, & Alraek, 2008)

Complete systematic review and protocol information may be accessed at www.cochrane.org/index.htm.

Examples of Clinical Trials

- L-Arginine Supplements in Women Who Are Cancer Survivors (No phase specified. Sponsors: Wake Forest University, NCI. Protocol IDs: CCCW-FU-05-04-0, CCCWFU-97106, WFU 05-04-01, NCT00459134. Active.)
- Can Hyperbaric Oxygen Improve Erectile Function Following Surgery for Prostate Cancer (HBOT) (Phase IV. Sponsor: Hartford Hospital. Protocol IDs: STAF001982HU, NCT00906269. Active.)
- Communication and Intimacy—Enhancing Therapy for Men With Early Stage Prostate Cancer and Their Partners (No phase specified. Sponsors: Memorial Sloan-Kettering Cancer Center, NCI. Protocol IDs: MSKCC-07069, 07-069, NCT00503646. Active.)

Complete clinical trial information may be accessed at http://cancer.gov/clinicaltrials.

Special Considerations

Pediatrics

Adolescents and young adults with cancer remain a unique challenge. These individuals may find it difficult to access appropriate sexual health knowledge, manage a changing body image, and effectively deal with interpersonal relationships (Krebs, 2010). Canada, Schover, and Li (2007) evaluated a program of two individual counseling sessions to enhance psychosexual development. Following the intervention, participants had increased knowledge and body image and decreased concerns about romantic and sexual relationships. These gains were maintained at three months following the intervention. Programs such as this need further evaluation but appear to be a good beginning for managing the unique issues of sexuality in adolescents and young adults with cancer.

Older Adults

Management of sexuality issues in older adults with cancer is complex. It includes integrating cancer, comorbidities, aging, partner availability, social isolation, and alterations in housing and lifestyle. Cancer-related changes in physical and mental conditions coupled with comorbidities such as arthritis or dementia can affect both an interest in and the ability to take part in sexual activities (Kagan, Holland, & Chalian, 2008). Advancing age does not equate with a lack of interest in sexual expression.

Gay, Lesbian, Bisexual, and Transgender Individuals

Few studies have specifically evaluated the impact of cancer on the sexuality of gay, lesbian, bisexual, and transgender (GLBT) individuals. Blank (2005) described the impact of prostate cancer on gay men, noting that ED can have very different implications for them. He also commented that most discussions of ED are focused on vaginal intercourse for those in long-standing, opposite-sex, partnered relationships. Blank also suggested that gay men may need different support services and evaluation of psychosexual needs—two services not always provided. Arena et al. (2007) evaluated lesbian and heterosexual women with breast cancer, identifying that lesbians had less disruption in sexual activity, had fewer sexual concerns, and were more likely to use their current support systems to effectively manage the cancer experience. They noted that further research is needed to understand differences and similarities in order to provide comprehensive care.

Terminally Ill Patients and Palliative Care

The factors that affect sexuality for terminally ill patients are essentially the same as for those going through cancer treatment, although the focus may be different and the potential for returning to normalcy no longer exists. Issues of privacy and the ability to lie with one another may be affected by moving to a healthcare facility or having family, friends, and providers coming in and out. Permission may need to be given to sexually active patients, and other methods of sexual expression may need to be explored. Comprehensive symptom management (e.g., for pain, nausea, difficulty breathing, vaginal dryness) and strategies to conserve energy are essential, whereas appropriate education, including contraceptive use, should be provided as appropriate. When death is imminent, the patient and partner should be encouraged to express intimacy in whatever way is possible and comfortable, including touching, kissing, and verbalization of endearments (Morriss & Pace, 2008; Shell, 2008).

Summary

Alterations in sexual function are common in patients with cancer and those undergoing cancer treatments. Some form of alteration in sexuality will occur at some point during the person's illness. With cancer survival rates improving, and with the understanding that sexual function is important to all individuals, it is essential that sexuality be assessed and evaluated prior to therapy and that appropriate interventions, using all possible conventional and CAM options, be implemented throughout treatment and during the follow-up period.

References

Albaugh, A., Kellogg-Spadt, S., Krebs, L.U., Lewis, J.H., & Kramer-Levien, D. (2009). Sexual function and sexual rehabilitation with genitourinary cancer. In J. Held-Warmkessel (Ed.), *Site-specific cancer series: Genitourinary cancers* (pp. 121–148). Pittsburgh, PA: Oncology Nursing Society.

Annon, J.S. (1974). *The behavioral treatment of sexual problems* (pp. 43–47). Honolulu, HI: Mercantile Printing.

Arena, P.L., Carver, C.S., Antoni, M.H., Weiss, S., Ironson, G., & Duran, R.E. (2007). Psychosocial responses to treatment for breast cancer among lesbian and heterosexual women. *Women and Health, 44*(2), 81–102.

Blank, T.O. (2005). Gay men and prostate cancer: Invisible diversity. *Journal of Clinical Oncology, 23*(12), 2593–2596.

Canada, A.L., Schover, L.R., & Li, Y. (2007). A pilot intervention to enhance psychosexual development in adolescents and young adults with cancer. *Pediatric Blood and Cancer, 49*(6), 824–828.

Davis, S., & Taylor, B. (2006). From PLISSIT to Ex-PLISSIT. In S. Davis (Ed.), *Rehabilitation: The use of theories and models in practice* (pp. 101–129). Edinburgh, Scotland: Elsevier Churchill Livingstone.

Denton, A.S., & Maher, J. (2003). Interventions for the physical aspects of sexual dysfunction in women following pelvic radiotherapy. *Cochrane Database of Systematic Reviews* 2003, Issue 1. Art. No.: CD003750. DOI: 10.1002/14651858.CD003570.

Flynn, P., Kew, F., & Kisely, S.R. (2009). Interventions for psychosexual dysfunction in women treated for gynaecological malignancy. *Cochrane Database of Systematic Reviews* 2009, Issue 2. Art. No.: CD004708. DOI: 10.1002/14651858.pub2.

Kagan, S.H., Holland, H., & Chalian, A.A. (2008). Sexual issues in special populations: Geriatric oncology—sexuality and older adults. *Seminars in Oncology Nursing, 24*(2), 120–126.

Katz, A. (2007). *Breaking the silence on cancer and sexuality: A handbook for healthcare providers.* Pittsburgh, PA: Oncology Nursing Society.

Krebs, L. (2006). What should I say? Talking with patients about sexuality issues. *Clinical Journal of Oncology Nursing, 10*(3), 313–315.

Krebs, L.U. (2008). Sexual assessment in cancer care: Concepts, methods and strategies for success. *Seminars in Oncology Nursing, 24*(2), 80–90.

Krebs, L.U. (2010). Sexual and reproductive dysfunction. In C.H. Yarbro, B.H. Gobel, & D. Wujcik (Eds.), *Cancer nursing: Principles and practice* (7th ed., pp. 879–911). Sudbury, MA: Jones and Bartlett.

Liu, J., Fei, Y., & Alraek, T. (2008). Acupuncture for the treatment of erectile dysfunction (Protocol). *Cochrane Database of Systematic Reviews* 2008, Issue 3. Art. No.: CD007241. DOI: 10.1002/14651858.CD007241.

Melnik, T., Soares, B., & Nasello, A.G. (2007). Psychosocial interventions for erectile dysfunction. *Cochrane Database of Systematic Reviews* 2007, Issue 3. Art. No.: CD004825. DOI: 10.1002/14651858.CD004825.

Mick, J., Hughes, M., & Cohen, M.Z. (2004). Using the BETTER model to assess sexuality. *Clinical Journal of Oncology Nursing, 8*(1), 84–86.

Miles, C., Candy, B., Jones, L., Williams, R., Tookman, A., & King, M. (2007). Interventions for sexual dysfunction following treatments for cancer. *Cochrane Database of Systematic Reviews* 2007, Issue 4. Art. No.: CD005540. DOI: 10.1002/14651858.pub2.

Morriss, B.B., & Pace, J.C. (2008). Sexuality. In P. Esper & K.K. Kuebler (Eds.), *Palliative practices from A–Z for the bedside clinician* (2nd ed., pp. 235–240). Pittsburgh, PA: Oncology Nursing Society.

National Cancer Institute. (2009, October). *Sexual and reproductive issues (PDQ®)*. Retrieved August 23, 2009, from http://www.cancer.gov/cancertopics/pdq/supportivecare/sexuality/health professional

National Cancer Institute Cancer Therapy Evaluation Program. (2009). *Common terminology criteria for adverse events* [v.4.02]. Retrieved August 10, 2009, from http://evs.nci.nih.gov/ftp1/CTCAE/CTCAE_4.02_2009-09-15_QuickReference_8.5x11.pdf

Natural Medicines Comprehensive Database. (n.d.-a). *Natural product effectiveness checker: Erectile dysfunction*. Retrieved August 22, 2009, from http://www.naturaldatabase.com

Natural Medicines Comprehensive Database. (n.d.-b). *Natural product effectiveness checker: Sexual dysfunction*. Retrieved August 22, 2009, from http://www.naturaldatabase.com

Natural Standard Database. (n.d.). *Sexuality, erectile dysfunction, libido*. Retrieved August 22, 2009, from http://www.naturalstandard.com

Shell, J.A. (2008). Sexual issues in the palliative care population. *Seminars in Oncology Nursing, 24*(2), 131–134.

Tierney, D.K. (2008). Sexuality: A quality-of-life issue for cancer survivors. *Seminars in Oncology Nursing, 24*(2), 71–79.

Taste Changes

Introduction

Dysgeusia is a disorder characterized by abnormal sensual experience with the taste of foodstuffs; it can be related to a decrease in the sense of smell (NCI, 2009). Taste changes may be correlated with the site or extent of the tumor and be reported even before the patient starts cancer treatment (Yamagata et al., 2003). Because taste and smell are closely associated with eating, it is not clear whether these changes occur as a result of the changes in perception in taste or smell. Patients undergoing radiation therapy experience a rapid loss of taste (hypogeusia) within the first weeks of treatment with nearly a total loss by the third or fourth week. Many patients show improvement within four months (Ripamonti et al., 1998). Because malnutrition and weight loss are common in patients with cancer, whether disease- or treatment-related, more attention to ameliorating this symptom may result in improved nutritional status and overall well-being.

Toxicity grading for this symptom according to the CTCAE (NCI CTEP, 2009) can be added to the clinical evaluation and reported in the medical record. The criteria range from altered taste alone (grade 1) to altered taste with change in diet or loss of taste (grade 2) (see Table 24).

Table 24. Common Terminology Criteria for Adverse Events: Dysgeusia					
Adverse Event	**Grade**				
	1	2	3	4	5
Dysgeusia	Altered taste but no change in diet	Altered taste with change in diet (e.g., oral supplements); noxious or unpleasant taste; loss of taste	–	–	–

Note. From *Common Terminology Criteria for Adverse Events* [v.4.02] (p. 52), by National Cancer Institute Cancer Therapy Evaluation Program, 2009. Retrieved November 23, 2009, from http://evs.nci.nih.gov/ftp1/CTCAE/CTCAE_4.02_2009-09-15_QuickReference_8.5x11.pdf.

Evidence for Practice

Although a wide range of interventions for the management of taste changes have been studied, evidence is limited, and treatment is mainly palliative. Successful conventional interventions are minimal to treat aspects of this symptom. Patients who choose to augment conventional approaches have several economical, safe, and effective CAM therapy options available.

Evidence	Natural Standard	Natural Medicines Comprehensive Database	Physician Data Query
Strong Scientific Evidence	• None at this time	• None at this time	• None at this time
Good to Moderate Scientific Evidence	• None at this time	• None at this time	• Zinc supplements
Weak, Negative, or Conflicting Scientific Evidence	• Zinc	• Zinc	• None at this time

Examples of Ongoing Science

Cochrane Collaboration Systematic Reviews

• None at this time

Cochrane Collaboration Protocols

• None at this time
  Complete systematic review and protocol information may be accessed at www.cochrane.org/index.htm.

Examples of Clinical Trials

• None at this time
  Complete clinical trial information may be accessed at http://cancer.gov/clinicaltrials.

Special Considerations

Pediatrics

The COG Nutrition Committee is furthering the knowledge of nutrition in children with cancer by education and the conduct of clinical trials. COG has developed an algorithm as a guideline for nutritional intervention (Children's Hospital of New York-Presbyterian, 2009).

Older Adults

Older patients experience a reduction in taste sensation and olfactory function but not taste discrimination. For example, older adults may be able to distinguish sweet from salty but may need to add more salt to food to taste it completely (American Geriatrics Society, 2009).

Summary

Patients undergoing treatment for cancer often report changes in their sense of taste. Conventional interventions ameliorating this symptom are safe and effective but may not be scientifically based. Taste perception is impaired temporarily and can be regenerated in most patients. Numerous self-help interventions are available to alleviate the severity but not the duration of taste changes in patients undergoing chemotherapy and radiation therapy. CAM interventions are emerging with a supportive scientific basis for incorporation into practice.

References

American Geriatrics Society. (2009). *Palliative care.* Retrieved August 20, 2009, from http://www.americangeriatrics.org

Children's Hospital of New York-Presbyterian. (2009). *The Integrative Therapies Program for Children With Cancer, 2009.* Retrieved August 20, 2009, from http://integrativetherapies.columbia.edu

National Cancer Institute. (2009, October). *Oral complications of chemotherapy and head/neck radiation (PDQ®): Taste dysfunction.* Retrieved September 8, 2009, from http://www.cancer.gov/cancertopics/pdq/supportivecare/oralcomplications/healthprofessional/allpages#Section_329

National Cancer Institute Cancer Treatment Evaluation Program. (2009). *Common terminology criteria for adverse events* [v.4.02]. Retrieved August 20, 2009, from http://evs.nci.nih.gov/ftp1/CTCAE/CTCAE_4.02_2009-09-15_QuickReference_8.5x11.pdf

Natural Medicines Comprehensive Database. (n.d.). *Natural product effectiveness checker: Anorexia.* Retrieved August 20, 2009, from http://www.naturaldatabase.com

Natural Standard Database. (n.d.). *Taste changes (cancer related).* Retrieved August 20, 2009, from http://www.naturalstandard.com

Ripamonti, C., Zecca, E., Brunelli, C., Fulfaro, F., Villa, S., Balzarini, A., et al. (1998). A randomized, controlled clinical trial to evaluate the effects of zinc sulfate on cancer patients with taste alterations caused by head and neck irradiation. *Cancer, 82*(10), 1938–1945.

Yamagata, T., Nakamura, Y., Yamagata, Y., Nakanishi, M., Matsunaga, K., Nakanishi, H., et al. (2003). The pilot trial of the prevention of the increase in electrical taste thresholds by zinc containing fluid infusion during chemotherapy to treat primary lung cancer. *Journal of Experimental and Clinical Cancer Research, 22*(4), 557–563.

Xerostomia

Introduction

Xerostomia is the subjective sensation of a dry mouth, usually the result of decreased volume of secreted saliva or a change in the composition of saliva (NCI, 2009). Salivary gland dysfunction is an umbrella term for both xerostomia and salivary gland hypofunction and is a predictable side effect of radiation therapy to the head and neck region. It develops soon after radiation therapy begins, progresses, and is essentially permanent. Among the symptoms associated with salivary hypofunction are oral discomfort, taste changes, difficulty chewing and swallowing, speech changes, dental caries, and oral candidiasis. Xerostomia may or may not occur in the presence of salivary gland hypofunction but usually is associated with a high level of morbidity in patients with advanced cancer (Davies, 1997).

Toxicity grading for this symptom according to the CTCAE (NCI CTEP, 2009) can be added to the clinical evaluation and reported in the medical record. The criteria range from symptomatic without significant dietary alteration (grade 1) to inability to adequately aliment orally and tube feeding or TPN indicated (grade 3) (see Table 25).

Adverse Event	Grade				
	1	2	3	4	5
Dry mouth	Symptomatic (dry or thick saliva) without significant dietary alteration; unstimulated saliva flow > 0.2 ml/min	Symptomatic and significant oral intake alteration (e.g., copious water, other lubricants, diet limited to purees and/or soft, moist foods); unstimulated saliva 0.1–0.2 ml/min	Inability to adequately aliment orally; tube feeding or TPN indicated; unstimulated saliva < 0.1 ml/min	–	–

Table 25. Common Terminology Criteria for Adverse Events: Dry Mouth

TPN—total parenteral nutrition

Note. From *Common Terminology Criteria for Adverse Events* [v.4.02] (p. 13), by National Cancer Institute Cancer Therapy Evaluation Program, 2009. Retrieved November 23, 2009, from http://evs.nci.nih.gov/ftp1/CTCAE/CTCAE_4.02_2009-09-15_QuickReference_8.5x11.pdf.

Evidence for Practice

Although a wide range of interventions for the management of xerostomia have been studied, evidence is limited, and treatment is mainly palliative. Successful conventional interventions are available. Patients who choose to augment conventional approaches have limited economical, safe, and effective CAM options available.

Evidence	Natural Standard	Natural Medicines Comprehensive Database	Physician Data Query
Strong Scientific Evidence	• None at this time	• None at this time	• None at this time
Good to Moderate Scientific Evidence	• None at this time	• None at this time	• None at this time
Weak, Negative, or Conflicting Scientific Evidence	• Acupuncture • Yohimbe bark extract	• None at this time	• Povidine-iodine oral rinses
Lack Sufficient Evidence	• Blessed thistle • Blue flag • Bovine colostrums • Canada balsam • Ginseng • Horseradish • Hydrangea • Quassia • Yerba santa	• None at this time	• None at this time

Examples of Ongoing Science

Cochrane Collaboration Systematic Reviews

• None at this time

Cochrane Collaboration Protocols

• None at this time

Complete systematic review and protocol information may be accessed at www.cochrane.org/index.htm.

Examples of Clinical Trials

- Electroacupuncture for Chronic Dry Mouth Caused by Radiation Therapy in Patients With Head and Neck Cancer (No phase specified. Supportive care. Sponsors: Mayo Clinic, NCI. Protocol IDs: MAYO-MC S285, NCT00623129. Active.)
- Acupuncture for Prevention of Radiation-Induced Xerostomia (No phase specified. Supportive care, treatment. Sponsors: M.D. Anderson Cancer Center, NCI. Protocol IDs: 2006-0763, NCT00430378. Active.)

Complete clinical trial information may be accessed at http://cancer.gov/clinicaltrials.

Special Considerations

Pediatrics

The COG Nutrition Committee is furthering the knowledge of nutrition in children with cancer by education and the conduct of clinical trials. COG has developed an algorithm as a guideline for nutritional intervention (Children's Hospital of New York-Presbyterian, 2009).

Older Adults

Salivary function is not noticeably reduced with aging, but xerostomia can be a common complaint of older adults, usually because of the adverse effects of medication (American Geriatrics Society, 2009).

Summary

Patients undergoing treatment for cancer often report xerostomia. Conventional interventions ameliorating this symptom are safe and effective. Numerous self-help interventions are available to alleviate the severity and duration of xerostomia in patients undergoing chemotherapy and/or radiation therapy. CAM interventions are emerging with a supportive scientific basis for incorporation into practice.

References

American Geriatrics Society. (2009). *Palliative care.* Retrieved August 20, 2009, from http://www.americangeriatrics.org/

Children's Hospital of New York-Presbyterian. (2009). *The Integrative Therapies Program for Children With Cancer, 2009.* Retrieved August 20, 2009, from http://integrativetherapies.columbia.edu

Davies, A.N. (1997). The management of xerostomia: A review. *European Journal of Cancer Care,* *6*(3), 209–214.

National Cancer Institute. (2009). *Oral complications of chemotherapy and head/neck radiation (PDQ®): Xerostomia.* Retrieved August 20, 2009 from http://www.cancer.gov/cancertopics/ pdq/supportivecare/oralcomplications/healthprofessional/allpages#Section_181

National Cancer Institute Cancer Therapy Evaluation Program. (2009). *Common terminology criteria for adverse events* [v.4.02]. Retrieved August 20, 2009, from http://evs.nci.nih.gov/ftp1/ CTCAE/CTCAE_4.02_2009-09-15_QuickReference_8.5x11.pdf

Natural Medicines Comprehensive Database. (2009). *Natural product effectiveness checker: Anorexia.* Retrieved August 20, 2009, from http://www.naturaldatabase.com

Natural Standard Database. (2009). *Dry mouth (cancer related).* Retrieved August 20, 2009, from http://www.naturalstandard.com

Nutritional Considerations

Introduction

Kogut and Luthringer (2005) framed the issues related to nutrition in symptom management, signifying that nutritional care is complex and therefore must be individualized in meeting the nutritional challenges of patients with cancer. The entire healthcare team has never been more important. It is not just the number of calories alone—nutrition (i.e., protein, fat, and carbohydrates) is important in patient care. Central to personalized nutritional intervention in oncology is assessment and determination of risk. The Patient-Generated Subjective Global Assessment (PG-SGA) offers nurses a validated, easy-to-use assessment tool (Ottery, 1996). Decker and Grant (2008) offered a method for nurses to determine nutritional risk and an appropriate intervention.

Low Risk

- PG-SGA score (0–3 points), institution-specific criteria, or low-risk considerations
- Interventions: patient and family education, general nutrition counseling, symptom management
- Reassessment every 14 days

Low-Risk Considerations

- Age: younger than age 65
- Comorbidities: none
- Cancer type: bladder, brain, breast, gynecologic, genitourinary, skin (excluding melanoma), sarcoma
- Cancer stage: stage I
- Food intake: good, no change in appetite
- Symptoms: none
- Change in weight: no change

Moderate Risk

- PG-SGA score (4–8 points), institution-specific criteria, or moderate-risk considerations
- Interventions: individualized nutrition counseling, symptom management
- Reassessment every seven days

Moderate-Risk Considerations

- Age: older than age 65
- Comorbidities: controlled
- Cancer type: central nervous system tumors, leukemia/lymphomas, liver, melanoma, myeloma, renal cell
- Cancer stage: stage II
- Food intake: fair; eats 50%–75% of meals or usual intake
- Symptoms: one to three symptoms (e.g., anorexia and mucositis)
- Change in weight: 5% weight loss within one month or 10% in six months

High Risk

- PG-SGA score (greater than 9 points), institution-specific criteria, or high-risk considerations.
- Interventions: patient and family education, individualized nutrition counseling, symptom management
- Reassessment every five days

High-Risk Considerations

- Age: older than age 80
- Comorbidities: uncontrolled
- Cancer type: colorectal, esophageal, gastric, head and neck, lung, pancreatic
- Cancer stage: stage III, IV
- Food intake: poor; eats less than 50% of meals or usual intake
- Symptoms: more than three symptoms
- Change in weight: more than 5% weight loss within one month or more than 10% in six months

Specific Interventions for Patients at High Risk

- Early intervention is key. Preventing malnutrition is easier and preferable to reversing it.
- Does the patient have cancer-induced weight loss? *These patients are most at risk for cachexia—use cancer-specific supplements and formulas.*

- Does the patient have weight loss associated with impaired intake? *Use intact protein oral supplements and formulas.*
- Does the patient have impaired digestion and absorption? *Use oral elemental and semi-elemental formulas.*
- Does the patient have surgical and wound-management concerns, infectious complications, or an increased risk for infection? *Use condition-specific oral supplements or formulas.*
- Does the patient have a bowel obstruction, short bowel syndrome, high-output fistula, severe radiation enteritis, diarrhea, or intractable nausea and vomiting refractory to medical intervention? *Oral or enteral formulas are contraindicated. Total parenteral nutrition (TPN) is indicated.*

Characterization of Nutritional Status

- Factors related to food
  - Diet history
  - Food preferences, intolerances, aversions, and allergies
  - Three-day food diary
  - Ability to obtain, purchase, and prepare food
- Physical examination
  - Current height and weight
  - Serial weights (usually at each visit)
  - Assessment of skin, hair, mouth, teeth, and general muscle tone
  - Anthropometric measurements—mid-arm muscle circumference, subscapular, and tricep skin folds
- Laboratory analysis (for patients undergoing biotherapy and chemotherapy)
  - Serum transferrin
  - Serum albumin
  - Serum prealbumin
  - Complete blood count with differential
  - Electrolytes, minerals, trace elements, and vitamins

Collaborative Management of Nutritional Needs

- Dietary or certified nutritionist consultation whenever possible
- High-calorie, high-protein supplements if indicated
- Pharmacologic intervention as appropriate
- Enteral nutrition if patient is not able to meet caloric requirements orally
- TPN if patient has altered GI function or is not able to tolerate enteral nutrition
- Introduction of community resources to assist with nutrition (e.g., Meals on Wheels)

Education of Patients and Families

- Perform oral care prior to mealtime.
- Monitor weight weekly.
- Eat small, frequent meals slowly.
- Incorporate high-protein foods, such as cheese, milk, eggs, beans, nuts, yogurt, and pudding.
- Marinate meats to enhance or disguise flavor.
- Avoid gas-forming foods—broccoli, cabbage, carbonated beverages.
- Drink fluids with meals but in moderate quantities.
- Avoid drinking large amounts of fluids, which may reduce intake of solid foods.
- Incorporate hard candy and fresh fruit to provide pleasant flavor.
- Plan daily food preparation to accommodate energy level.
- Avoid smoking, which may affect sense of smell and taste.
- Alter food preparation plans for variety: takeout, frozen dinners, new recipes, freezing small portions.
- Engage in mild exercise for 15–20 minutes daily to stimulate muscles and increase strength.
- Avoid spicy, coarse, hot, cold, or acidic foods, juices, and medications, as well as beverages containing alcohol.
- Incorporate soft, moist foods and nonalcoholic beverages.

Summary

Nutritional assessment is indicated for all patients with cancer. Although the participation of the healthcare team is ideal, it is not always possible. For some patients, weight gain can negatively affect prognosis as significantly as weight loss can for others. Serial weight assessment provides a simple yet essential cornerstone in identifying potential nutritional deficiencies. Completion of nutritional self-assessment tools like the PG-SGA help to create a partnership and provide patients an opportunity to participate with their HCPs in a plan of care. It is no longer acceptable to instruct a patient to eat just anything. Patients with cancer require nutrition—protein, fat, and carbohydrates. The role of nutrition in integrative oncology continues to unfold.

References

Decker, G., & Grant, B. (2008). *Nutritional challenges in oncology: Keys to optimizing patient outcomes.* Retrieved August 20, 2009, from http://www.ons.org/cecentral/more/webcasts.shtml

Kogut, V.J., & Luthringer, S.L. (Eds.). (2005). *Nutritional issues in cancer care.* Pittsburgh, PA: Oncology Nursing Society.

Ottery, F.D. (1996). Definition of standardized nutritional assessment and interventional pathways in oncology. *Nutrition, 12*(Suppl. 1), S15–S19.

CAM Regulation and Adverse Event Reporting

Regulation: Dietary Supplements and Devices

Dietary Supplement Health and Education Act of 1994

For CAM therapies that are not provider-based, such as nutritional therapies or dietary supplements, the FDA gives oversight through the Dietary Supplement Health and Education Act (DSHEA) of 1994 (FDA, 2009a). Prior to 1994, supplements were not regulated; rather, they were marketed either as foods or as drugs, depending on their intended use and claims. The DSHEA allows manufacturers to use various statements on a product label that do not need preapproval, although claims must not be made about the diagnosis, prevention, treatment, or cure for a specific disease. The labeling of these items must remain void of this information at all times.

The DSHEA grants the FDA the authority to develop good manufacturing practices governing preparation, packing, and holding of products (FDA, 2009a). The NIH Office of Dietary Supplements (n.d.) also was created as a result of the DSHEA to promote, collect, and compile research and to maintain a database on supplements and individual nutrients. From a consumer standpoint, the DSHEA allows for over-the-counter access to an array of products without the prerequisite of stringent requirement on manufacturing, product characterization, safety and efficacy data, and benefit claim as required for conventional medicines (Kinsel & Straus, 2003).

Federal Food, Drug, and Cosmetic Act of 1938 (Amended 2004)

CAM providers are becoming more cognizant of the federal government's requirement for approval of any medical devices used in the treatment of patients. The FDA's legal authority to regulate both medical devices and electronic radiation-emitting products is the Federal Food, Drug, and Cosmetic Act (FDA, 2009b). FDA's Center for Devices and Radiological Health (CDRH) is responsible for "regulating firms who manufacture, repackage, relabel, and/or import medical devices sold in the United States" (FDA, 2009c). In addition, CDRH regulates radiation-emitting electronic medical and nonmedical products such as lasers, x-ray and ultrasound equipment, microwaves, and televisions. Examples of CAM devices that are currently under regulatory authority of the FDA are acupuncture needles and acupressure bands.

MedWatch: The FDA Safety Information and Adverse Event Reporting System

MedWatch is a program that provides new safety information on drugs, devices, dietary supplements, and cosmetics (Marks, 2009). Alerts in the form of e-mails and postings on the Web site contain information about adverse events and the need to monitor patients closely and make any necessary adjustments. This timely information can avert unnecessary harm, allow the intervention to continue to be used safely, and lead to better health outcomes. When a problem is reported to the FDA, the following review is completed:

- Is an illness or injury involved? If so, what is the health hazard?
- Is the illness possibly an allergic reaction to a food or a drug or, in the case of drugs, is it a reaction already known to occur with that product?
- Is the problem life threatening?
- Is the product likely to be associated with the problem?
- Is the problem likely to be widespread, or is this an isolated case?
- Is more information needed about the problem or the product?
- Is the product or problem within the jurisdiction of the FDA, or is it the responsibility of another federal agency or local or state government?

The FDA receives more than 40,000 adverse event reports directly from doctors, other clinicians, and their patients. Hundreds of thousands of similar reports sent from clinicians to manufacturers are received indirectly by the FDA. Depending on the seriousness of the problem, the FDA will either investigate it immediately or will cover it during the next inspection of the facility responsible for the product. To report an adverse event online, the MedWatch Online Voluntary Reporting Form (www.accessdata.fda.gov/scripts/medwatch/medwatch-online.htm) is used.

References

Kinsel, J.F., & Straus, S.E. (2003). Complementary and alternative therapeutics: Rigorous research is needed to support claims. *Annual Review of Pharmacology and Toxicology, 43,* 463–484.

Marks, N.S. (2009, March). *MedWatch: Safety information and adverse event reporting.* Retrieved August 29, 2009, from http://cme.medscape.com/viewarticle/588757

National Institutes of Health Office of Dietary Supplements. (n.d.). *About the Office of Dietary Supplements.* Retrieved January 23, 2007, from http://dietary-supplements.info.nih.gov/About/about_ods.aspx

U.S. Food and Drug Administration. (2009a, May). *Dietary Supplement Health and Education Act of 1994.* Retrieved August 29, 2009, from http://www.fda.gov/RegulatoryInformation/Legislation/FederalFoodDrugandCosmeticActFDCAct/SignificantAmendmentstotheFDCAct/ucm148003.htm

U.S. Food and Drug Administration. (2009b, September). *Federal Food, Drug, and Cosmetic Act: Regulatory information.* Retrieved August 29, 2009, from http://www.fda.gov/Regulatory Information/Legislation/FederalFoodDrugandCosmeticActFDCAct/defautt.htm

U.S. Food and Drug Administration. (2009c, November). *Overview of device regulation.* Retrieved August 29, 2009, from http://www.fda.gov/MedicalDevices/DeviceRegulationandGuidance/ Overview/default.htm

Glossary of Terms

alternative therapy. Therapies used in place of conventional medicine (NCCAM, 2007).

American Botanical Council. Independent, nonprofit research and educational organization dedicated to providing reliable information to healthcare providers, consumers, educators, industry, researchers, and media (American Botanical Council, n.d.).

American Cancer Society. National, community-based voluntary health organization dedicated to eliminating cancer as a major health problem by preventing cancer and diminishing suffering through research, education, services, and advocacy (ACS, n.d.-b).

American Holistic Nurses Association. Nonprofit membership association for nurses and other holistic HCPs dedicated to promoting holistic nursing and education in holistic caring and healing (AHNA, n.d.).

animal assisted therapy. Therapy in which pets visit people; more specifically, a therapy directed and delivered by an HCP or human service professional with specialized expertise to promote improvement in human physical, social, or cognitive function (Delta Society, n.d.).

aromatherapy. Refers to several modalities that deliver essential oils to the body. Essential oils are mixed with carrier oil or diluted in alcohol before being applied to the skin, sprayed in the air, or inhaled. Massage is a common means of delivering oils into the body through the skin (ACS, 2008).

art therapy. A variety of art-based assessments that are used clinically and in research based on the belief that the creative process of art is both healing and life enhancing. Art therapists use drawing, painting, and other art-based techniques to assess and treat clients with emotional, cognitive, physical, and developmental needs (American Art Therapy Association, n.d.).

Ayurveda. Vedic word *Ayurveda* (*ayu* and *veda*) means "life" and "science." According to Ayurveda medicine, every human body is governed by three principles called doshas, derived from the five elements: Vata (space and air), Pitha (fire and water), and Kapha (water and earth), and the Ayurvedic recommendations vary according to doshas. Ayurvedic herbs are concentrated with biologically active compounds naturally found in plants called phytochemicals (Manek, n.d.).

chiropractic medicine. Healthcare profession that focuses on disorders of the musculoskeletal and nervous systems and the impact of disorders in these systems on individual general health. Chiropractic care is used often to treat neuromusculoskeletal complaints, including back pain, neck pain, joint pain, and headaches (American Chiropractic Association, n.d.).

complementary and alternative medicine. Group of diverse medical and healthcare systems, practices, and products thought to be used outside of conventional medicine (NCCAM, 2007).

complementary therapy. Therapy that is used together with conventional medicine (NCCAM, 2007).

conventional therapy. Currently accepted and widely used treatment for a certain type of disease, based on the results of past research, also referred to as conventional treatment (NCI, n.d.).

Dietary Supplement Health and Education Act (DSHEA). For CAM therapies that are not provider-based, such as nutritional therapies or dietary supplements, the U.S. Food and Drug Administration gives oversight through the DSHEA of 1994. DSHEA allows manufacturers to use various statements on a product label that do not need preapproval, although claims must not be made about the diagnosis, prevention, treatment, or cure for a specific disease. The labeling of these items must remain void of this information at all times (FDA, 2009b).

end-of-life care. When a patient and the patient's healthcare team determine that the cancer can no longer be controlled, medical testing and cancer treatment often stop, and the patient's care continues elsewhere. The care focuses on making the patient comfortable, as each individual has unique needs for information and support. The end of life is different for each person, and the patient's and family's questions and concerns should be discussed with the healthcare team as they arise (NCI, 2002).

folk medicine. Healing practices widely known to much of the population in a culture, stated informally as general knowledge and practice. This knowledge and practice can be applied by anyone in the culture (http://en.wikipedia.org/wiki/Folk_medicine).

U.S. Food and Drug Administration (FDA). Agency within the U.S. Department of Health and Human Services that consists of centers and offices responsible for protecting the public health by ensuring the safety, efficacy, and security of human and veterinary drugs, biologic products, medical devices, the nation's food supply, cosmetics, and products that emit radiation (FDA, 2009a).

healing touch. Relaxing energy therapy that uses gentle touch to balance physical, mental, emotional, and spiritual well-being. Healing touch works with an energy field to support natural ability to heal and is safe for all ages and works in harmony with standard medical care (Healing Touch International, n.d.).

homeopathy. System of medicine based on three principles: (a) like cures like: If the symptoms of your cold are similar to poisoning by mercury, then mercury would be your homeopathic remedy; (b) minimal dose: The remedy is taken in an extremely dilute form; normally one part of the remedy to around 1,000,000,000,000 parts of water; and (c) the single remedy: No matter how many symptoms are experienced, only one remedy is taken, and that remedy will be aimed at all those symptoms (ABC Homeopathy, n.d.).

hydropathy. Therapeutic system that professes to cure all disease with water, either by bathing in it or by drinking it (Hydrotherapy, 2009).

integrative medicine. Medicine that combines treatments from conventional medicine and CAM for which evidence of safety and effectiveness is available. Informed by evidence, integrative medicine uses therapeutic approaches to attain optimal health and healing and strives to achieve wholeness and health in addition to curing illness and disease (Bravewell Collaborative, n.d.).

integrative oncology. Expansion of conventional cancer care that includes mind, body, soul, and spirit; renews focus of medicine to include foundational principles; includes translational, preventive, and supportive care medicine; and develops recommendations based on therapy goals and an individualized risk-benefit analysis (Mumber, 2006).

investigational treatment/drug. Substance that has been tested in a laboratory and is approved by the FDA to be tested in humans for use in one disease or condition but may be considered investigational in other diseases or conditions (NCI, n.d.).

music therapy. Therapy that uses music to address physical, emotional, cognitive, and social needs of individuals of all ages. Music therapy interventions can be designed to promote wellness, manage stress, alleviate pain, express feelings, enhance memory, improve communication, and promote physical rehabilitation (American Music Therapy Association, n.d.).

National Center for Complementary and Alternative Medicine (NCCAM). Center within the National Institutes of Health (NIH) dedicated to research on the diverse medical and healthcare systems, practices, and products associated with CAM. NCCAM's efforts cross over disease types and NIH institutes, one of which is cancer (NCCAM, 2009).

NCCAM Backgrounder. Series of education documents developed by NCCAM on CAM modalities and use and efficacy, safety, and research areas designed to provide detailed information to HCPs and consumers (http://nccam.nih.gov/health/atoz.htm).

Office of Cancer Complementary and Alternative Medicine (OCCAM). Office within the NCI established in 1998 to coordinate and enhance the activities of the NCI in CAM as it related to cancer prevention, diagnosis, treatment, and symptom management (OCCAM, 2009).

Oncology Nursing Society. Oncology professional organization with more than 37,000 RNs and other HCPs dedicated to excellence in patient care, education, research, and administration in oncology nursing (Oncology Nursing Society, n.d.).

osteopathy. Whole system approach to health care that treats specific symptoms but with a major concentration on the individual as a whole person, focusing special attention on the musculoskeletal system (American Osteopathic Association, n.d.).

palliative care. Care designed to relieve the pain, symptoms, and stress of serious illness regardless of the prognosis. It is appropriate for people of any age and at any point in an illness. It can be delivered along with curative treatments typically provided by a team that includes palliative care doctors, nurses, and social workers working in partnership with a primary provider (Center to Advance Palliative Care, n.d.).

Physician Data Query (PDQ®). NCI's comprehensive cancer database containing peer-reviewed summaries on cancer treatment, screening, prevention, genetics, and supportive care and CAM. PDQ also maintains a registry of more than 8,000 open and 19,000 closed cancer clinical trials from around the world in addition to a directory of professionals who provide genetic services (NCI, 2009).

quackery. A type of approach to medical care that is derived from the word *quacksalver* (someone who boasts about his salves). It can also be known as a pretender or a charlatan. Many promoters sincerely believe in what they are doing (Barrett, 2009).

quality of life. Refers to the overall enjoyment of life. Many clinical trials assess the effects of cancer and its treatment on individuals' quality of life, measuring aspects of individuals' sense of well-being and ability to carry out various activities (NCI, n.d.).

unproven therapy. Any therapy that has not been scientifically tested and approved, including therapies that are under investigation (ACS, n.d.-a).

References

ABC Homeopathy. (n.d.). *What are homeopathics?* Retrieved November 19, 2009, from http://abchomeopathy.com/homeopathy.htm

American Art Therapy Association. (n.d.). *About art therapy.* Retrieved November 19, 2009, from http://www.americanarttherapyassociation.org/aata-aboutarttherapy.html

American Botanical Council. (n.d.). *About the American Botanical Council.* Retrieved November 18, 2009, from http://abc.herbalgram.org/site/PageServer?pagename=About_Us

American Cancer Society. (2008, November). *Aromatherapy.* Retrieved November 18, 2009, from http://www.cancer.org/docroot/ETO/content/ETO_5_3X_Aromatherapy.asp?sitearea=ETO

American Cancer Society. (n.d.-a). *Glossary search.* Retrieved November 19, 2009, from http://www.cancer.org/docroot/gry/gry_0.asp?txtSearch=unproven+therapy&dictionary=&btnGo.x=14&btnGo.y=7

American Cancer Society. (n.d.-b). *Who we are.* Retrieved November 18, 2009, from http://www.cancer.org/docroot/AA/AA_1.asp

American Chiropractic Association. (n.d.). *What is chiropractic?* Retrieved November 19, 2009, from http://www.acatoday.org/level2_css.cfm?T1ID=13&T2ID=61

American Holistic Nurses Association. (n.d.). *Welcome.* Retrieved November 18, 2009, from http://www.ahna.org

American Music Therapy Association. (n.d.). *What is music therapy?* Retrieved November 19, 2009, from http://www.musictherapy.org

American Osteopathic Association. (n.d.). *Osteopathic medicine.* Retrieved November 19, 2009, from http://www.osteopathic.org/index.cfm?PageID=ost_omed

Barrett, S. (2009, January). *Quackery: How should it be defined?* Retrieved November 19, 2009, from http://www.quackwatch.com/01QuackeryRelatedTopics/quackdef.html

Bravewell Collaborative. (n.d.). *Integrative medicine.* Retrieved November 19, 2009, from http://www.bravewell.org/integrative_medicine

Center to Advance Palliative Care. (n.d.). *What is palliative care?* Retrieved November 19, 2009, from http://www.getpalliativecare.org/whatis

Delta Society. (n.d.). *What are animal-assisted activities/therapy?* Retrieved November 18, 2009, from http://www.deltasociety.org/Document.Doc?id=10

Healing Touch International. (n.d.). *What is healing touch?* Retrieved November 19, 2009, from http://www.healingtouchinternational.org/index.php?option=com_content&task=view&id=2&Itemid=240

Hydropathy. (2009). In *Encyclopædia Britannica.* Retrieved November 19, 2009, from http://www.britannica.com/EBchecked/topic/278959/hydropathy

Manek, M. (n.d.). *Definition of Ayurvedic body typing video.* Retrieved November 19, 2009, from http://www.healthynewage.com/blog/ayurvedic-body-type

Mumber, M.P. (2006). Principles of integrative oncology. In M.P. Mumber (Ed.), *Integrative oncology principles and practice* (pp. 3–15). New York: Taylor and Francis.

National Cancer Institute. (2002, October). *National Cancer Institute fact sheet. End-of-life care: Questions and answers.* Retrieved November 19, 2009, from http://www.nci.nih.gov/cancertopics/factsheet/Support/end-of-life-care

National Cancer Institute. (2009, May). *PDQ®—NCI's Comprehensive Cancer Database.* Retrieved November 19, 2009, from http://www.cancer.gov/cancertopics/pdq/cancerdatabase

National Cancer Institute. (n.d.). *Dictionary of cancer terms.* Retrieved November 19, 2009, from http://nci.nih.gov/dictionary

National Center for Complementary and Alternative Medicine. (2007, February). *What is CAM?* Retrieved November 18, 2009, from http://nccam.nih.gov/health/whatiscam/overview.htm

National Center for Complementary and Alternative Medicine. (2009, August). *About NCCAM.* Retrieved November 19, 2009, from http://nccam.nih.gov/about

Office of Cancer Complementary and Alternative Medicine. (2009, October). *About us.* Retrieved November 19, 2009, from http://www.cancer.gov/cam/about_us.html

Oncology Nursing Society. (n.d.). *About ONS.* Retrieved November 19, 2009, from http://www.ons.org/about

U.S. Food and Drug Administration. (2009a, September). *About FDA: Centers and offices.* Retrieved November 19, 2009, from http://www.fda.gov/AboutFDA/CentersOffices/default.htm

U.S. Food and Drug Administration. (2009b, September). *Legislation.* Retrieved November 19, 2009, from http://www.fda.gov/opacom/laws/dshea.html

Society for Integrative Oncology Evidence-Based Clinical Practice Guidelines for Integrative Oncology

Complementary and Alternative Therapies Recommendations
Complementary and Alternative Therapies Recommendations: The Clinical Encounter   *Advantages: Good clinical practice*   *Limitations: None*

1	Inquire about the use of complementary and alternative therapies as a routine part of initial evaluation of cancer patients. *Grade of recommendation: 1C*
2	All patients with cancer should receive guidance about the advantages and limitations in an open, evidence-based, and patient-centered manner by a qualified professional. Patients should be fully informed of the treatment approach, the nature of the specific therapies, potential risks and benefits, and realistic expectations. *Grade of recommendation: 1C*

Mind-Body Medicine Recommendations   *Advantages: Safe, good evidence*   *Limitations: Time consuming*

3	Mind-body modalities are recommended as part of a multidisciplinary approach to reduce anxiety, mood disturbance, chronic pain, and improve quality of life. *Grade of recommendation: 1B*
4	Support groups, supportive and expressive therapy, cognitive-behavioral therapy, and cognitive-behavioral stress management are recommended as part of multidisciplinary approach to reduce anxiety, mood disturbance, chronic pain, and improve quality of life. *Grade of recommendation: 1A*

Manipulative and Body-Based Practice Recommendations   *Advantages: Safe, skills readily available*   *Limitations: None*

5	For patients with cancer experiencing anxiety or pain, massage therapy delivered by an oncology-trained massage therapist is recommended as part of multimodality treatment. *Grade of recommendation: 1C*

(Continued on next page)

Complementary and Alternative Therapies Recommendations *(Continued)*

| 6 | The application of deep or intense pressure is not recommended near cancer lesions or enlarged lymph nodes, radiation field sites, medical devices (such as indwelling intravenous catheters), or anatomic distortions such as postoperative changes or in patients with a bleeding tendency. *Grade of recommendation: 2B* |

Exercise and Physical Activity Recommendations
Advantages: Safe, good evidence
Limitations: None

| 7 | Regular physical activities can play many positive roles in cancer care. Patients should be referred to a qualified exercise specialist for guidelines on physical activity to promote basic health. *Grade of recommendation: 1B (1A for breast cancer survivors post-therapy for quality of life)* |
| 8 | Therapies based on a philosophy of bioenergy fields are safe and may provide some benefit for reducing stress and enhancing quality of life. The evidence is limited as to their efficacy for symptom management, including reducing pain and fatigue. *Grade of recommendation: 1B for reducing anxiety; 1C for pain, fatigue, and other symptom management* |

Acupuncture Recommendations
Advantages: Good evidence
Limitations: Skills not always readily available

9	Acupuncture is recommended as a complementary therapy when pain is poorly controlled, when nausea and vomiting associated with chemotherapy or surgical anesthesia are poorly controlled, or when the side effects from other modalities are clinically significant. *Grade of recommendation: 1A*
10	Acupuncture is recommended as a complementary therapy for radiation-induced xerostomia. *Grade of recommendation: 1B*
11	Acupuncture does not appear to be more effective than sham acupuncture for treatment of vasomotor symptoms (hot flashes) in postmenopausal women in general. In patients experiencing severe symptoms not amenable to pharmacologic treatment, however, a trial of acupuncture treatment for cancer can be considered. *Grade of recommendation: 1B*
12	For patients who do not stop smoking despite use of other options or those suffering from symptoms such as cancer-related dyspnea, cancer-related fatigue, chemotherapy-induced neuropathy, or post-thoracotomy pain, a trial of acupuncture may be helpful, but more clinical studies of acupuncture are warranted. *Grade of recommendation: 2C*
13	Acupuncture should be performed only by qualified practitioners and used cautiously in patients with bleeding tendencies. *Grade of recommendation: 1C*

(Continued on next page)

Complementary and Alternative Therapies Recommendations *(Continued)*

Diet Recommendations
Advantages: Interest the most patients
Limitations: Potential adverse effects

14	Research in diet and cancer prevention is based mainly on studies of populations consuming dietary components in whole-food form, with secure food supplies and access to a variety of food and drinks. Therefore, nutritional adequacy should be met by selecting a wide variety of foods; dietary supplements are usually unnecessary. *Grade of recommendation: 1B*
15	It is recommended that patients be advised regarding proper nutrition to promote basic health. *Grade of recommendation: 1B*
16	Based on current review of the literature, specific dietary supplements are not recommended for cancer prevention. *Grade of recommendation: 1A*
17	Evaluation of patients' use of dietary supplements prior to the start of cancer treatment is recommended. Also recommended is the referral of patients with cancer to trained professionals for guidelines on diets, nutritional supplementation, promotion of optimum nutritional status, management of tumor- and treatment-related symptoms, satisfaction of increased nutritional needs, and correction of any nutritional deficits while on active treatment. *Grade of recommendation: 1B*
18	It is recommended that dietary supplements, including botanicals and megadoses of vitamins and minerals, be evaluated for possible side effects and potential interaction with other drugs. Those that are likely to interact adversely with other drugs, including chemotherapeutic agents, should not be used concurrently with immunotherapy, chemotherapy, or radiation or prior to surgery. *Grade of recommendation: 1B*
19	For patients with cancer who wish to use nutritional supplements, including botanicals for purported antitumor effects, it is recommended that they consult a trained professional. During the consultation, the professional should provide support, discuss realistic expectations, and explore potential benefits and risks. It is recommended that use of those agents occur only in the context of clinical trials, recognized nutritional guidelines, clinical evaluation of the risk/benefit ratio based on available evidence, and close monitoring of adverse effects. *Grade of recommendation: 1C*
20	As with nutritional supplementation during treatment, survivors should be evaluated for supplement use and referred to a trained professional for evaluation to meet specific nutritional needs and to correct nutritional deficit as indicated. For older cancer survivors, nutritional supplementation may reduce nutrient inadequacies, although survivors who use supplements are usually the least likely to need them. *Grade of recommendation: 2B*

(Continued on next page)

Grading Recommendations *(Continued)*

Grade of Recommendation/ Description	Benefit Versus Risk and Burdens	Methodological Quality of Supporting Evidence	Implications
1A/strong recommendation, high-quality evidence	Benefits clearly outweigh risk and burdens, or vice versa	RCTs without important limitations or overwhelming evidence from observational studies	Strong recommendation, can apply to most patients in most circumstances without reservation
1B/strong recommendation, moderate-quality evidence	Benefits clearly outweigh risk and burdens, or vice versa	RCTs with important limitations (inconsistent results, methodological flaws, indirect, or imprecise) or exceptionally strong evidence from observational studies	Strong recommendation, can apply to most patients in most circumstances without reservation
1C/strong recommendation, low-quality or very low-quality evidence	Benefits clearly outweigh risk and burdens, or vice versa	Observational studies or case series	Strong recommendation but may change when higher quality evidence becomes available
2A/weak recommendation, high-quality evidence	Benefits closely balanced with risks and burden	RCTs without important limitations or overwhelming evidence from observational studies	Weak recommendation, best action may differ depending on circumstances or patients' or societal values
2B/weak recommendation, moderate-quality evidence	Benefits closely balanced with risks and burden	RCTs with important limitations (inconsistent results, methodological flaws, indirect, or imprecise) or exceptionally strong evidence from observational studies	Weak recommendation, best action may differ depending on circumstances or patients' or societal values

(Continued on next page)

Grading Recommendations *(Continued)*

Grade of Recommendation/ Description	Benefit Versus Risk and Burdens	Methodological Quality of Supporting Evidence	Implications
2C/weak recommendation, low-quality or very low-quality evidence	Uncertainty in the estimates of benefits, risks, and burden; benefits, risk, and burden may be closely balanced	Observational studies or case series	Very weak recommendations, other alternatives may be equally reasonable

RCTs—randomized controlled trials

Note. From "Evidence-Based Clinical Practice Guidelines for Integrative Oncology: Complementary Therapies and Botanicals," by G.E. Deng, M. Frenkel, L. Cohen, B.R. Cassileth, D.I. Abrams, J.L. Capodice, et al., 2009, *Journal of the Society for Integrative Oncology, 7*(3), pp. 85–120. Copyright 2009 by Society for Integrative Oncology. Reprinted with permission.

APPENDIX III

Oncology Nursing Society Position: The Use of Complementary and Alternative Therapies in Cancer Care

Complementary, alternative, and integrative therapies are healthcare systems, practices, and products not considered a part of conventional medicine. Complementary therapies are used concurrently with conventional medicine, alternative therapies are used in place of conventional medicine, and integrative therapies combine mainstream medical therapies with complementary or alternative therapies for which some high-quality scientific evidence of safety and efficacy exists (National Center for Complementary and Alternative Medicine, 2009).

In the United States, about 4 in 10 adults and 1 in 9 children are using some form complementary, alternative, or integrative therapy according to the National Health Interview Survey (Barnes, Bloom, & Nahim, 2008). These therapies have been broadly categorized as alternative medical systems, energy therapies, exercise therapies, manipulative and body-based methods, mind-body interventions, nutritional therapeutics, pharmacologic and biologic treatments, and spiritual therapies (Office of Cancer Complementary and Alternative Medicine, 2009). Non-vitamin, non-mineral natural products are the most commonly used complementary, alternative, or integrative therapies among adults. Use has increased for many therapies, including meditation, massage therapy, deep breathing exercises, and yoga (Barnes et al.). The list of therapies will likely continue to evolve as novel approaches are proven to be safe and effective, accepted as mainstream medicine, and integrated into cancer care.

Researchers report that patients with cancer and survivors are more likely to use these therapies than those without cancer (Basch & Ulbricht, 2004; Fouladbakhsh & Stommel, 2008). The most common reason for using them is a strong belief in their efficacy (Verhoef, Balneaves, Boon, & Vroegindewey, 2005). Methodologically rigorous preclinical and clinical research continues in the effort to establish safety and efficacy of these therapies through government and nongovernment funding sources. A clinical challenge is that 40%–77% of use remains undisclosed because of patients' beliefs that these therapies are natural and safe to use, concern that providers may react negatively, or simply, providers do not ask about their use (Robinson & McGrail, 2004).

Oncology nurses may be caring for patients without knowledge of concurrent complementary, alternative, and/or integrative therapy use. Routine assessment of use and close monitoring of patients using these therapies have the potential to enhance patient safety and promote integrative care (Lee, 2004).

It Is the Position of ONS That

- Oncology nurses evaluate their personal and professional beliefs regarding the use of complementary, alternative, and integrative therapies and recognize how these values can affect the care of patients seeking or using these therapies.
- Oncology nurses assess patients for the use of these therapies and provide evidence-based information and resources as well as information about verifying practitioners' qualifications and credentials.
- Oncology nurses have an awareness of the differences among terms applied to complementary, alternative, and integrative therapies and use the terms with consistency and in an appropriate context.
- Formal cancer education programs in schools of nursing and continuing education platforms include reliable information and access to learning about the therapies and promote integrated education with other health disciplines.
- Oncology nurses develop an awareness of complementary, alternative, and integrative therapies that potentially can interfere with the outcome of other cancer treatments.
- Oncology nurses document patients' use of and potential response to complementary, alternative, and integrative therapies.
- Oncology nurses seek proper training and obtain necessary credentials if practicing with complementary, alternative, and integrative therapies.
- Oncology nurses develop a working knowledge of cost reimbursement, liability, ethical, and legal issues surrounding complementary, alternative, and integrative therapies use in oncology care.
- Oncology nurses establish evidence-based practice in these areas by synthesizing present knowledge with regard to safety, efficacy, concurrent use with conventional therapy, and long-term use.
- ONS and its affiliates promote funding and collaboration in the design of methodologically rigorous treatment and supportive care clinical trials to study the impact of complementary, alternative, and integrative therapies on cancer care outcomes.

References

Barnes, P.M., Bloom, B., & Nahin, R. (2008). *National health statistics reports: Complementary and alternative medicine use among adults and children: United States, 2007.* Retrieved December 10, 2008, from http://www.cdc.gov/nchs/data/nhsr/nhsr012.pdf

Basch, E., & Ulbricht, C. (2004). Prevalence of CAM use among U.S. cancer patients: An update [Editorial]. *Journal of Cancer Integrative Medicine, 2*(1), 13–14.

Fouladbakhsh, J.M., & Stommel, M. (2008). Comparative analysis of CAM use in the U.S. cancer and noncancer populations. *Journal of Complementary and Integrative Medicine, 5*(1), 1–23.

Lee, C.O. (2004). Clinical trials in cancer part II. Biomedical, complementary, and alternative medicine: Significant issues. *Clinical Journal of Oncology Nursing, 8*(6), 670–674.

National Center for Complementary and Alternative Medicine. (2009). *What is CAM?* Retrieved February 3, 2009, from http://nccam.nih.gov/health/whatiscam/overview.htm

Office of Cancer Complementary and Alternative Medicine. (2009). *Categories of CAM therapies.* Retrieved February 3, 2009, from http://www.cancer.gov/CAM/health_categories.html

Robinson, A., & McGrail, M.R. (2004). Disclosure of CAM use to medical practitioners: A review of qualitative and quantitative studies. *Complementary Therapies in Medicine, 12*(2–3), 90–98.

Verhoef, M.J., Balneaves, L.G., Boon, H.S., & Vroegindewey, A. (2005). Reasons for and characteristics associated with complementary and alternative medicine use among adult cancer patients: A systematic review. *Integrative Cancer Therapies, 4*(4), 274–286.

Approved by the ONS Board of Directors 04/00; revised 06/02, 10/04, 03/06, 3/09.

The Ten Cardinal Rules of Herb Use

Research has shown that patients equate *natural* with *safe,* and some may believe that herbs are organ specific. For example, if antioxidants are used for cardiovascular health, patients may assume that they would not alter cancer therapy. This column is meant to be used as a teaching aid in improving communication between practitioners and patients.

Rule 1: Herbs should not be taken at the same time as any medicine. Taking herbs with prescription medicine or over-the-counter medicine changes the action of one or both.

Rule 2: "When in doubt, do without." If you experience an unpleasant side effect while taking an herb, discontinue immediately. Remember that the so-called "healing crisis" could, in fact, be life threatening.

Rule 3: Learn about herbs before using them. Do not take the advice of people who are not knowledgeable about medicine and herbs.

Rule 4: Accurate diagnosis is essential before using *any* therapy. Many factors should be considered before attempting self-treatment. Do you know or think you know your diagnosis? Guesswork should not be your guide.

Rule 5: Herbal medicines are medicines and should be treated as such. Treat herbal preparations with the same respect you would treat any medicine.

Rule 6: Some herbs are contraindicated in particular health situations. For example, some herbs cause low blood sugar and should not be used by those with hypoglycemia or hyperglycemia (diabetes), and others may alter blood-clotting mechanisms and should be avoided by people taking anticlotting medicines.

Rule 7: Herbs must be taken in specific doses at specific times. For example:
- Vitality and nutrition herbs and herbal formulas are best taken with meals.
- Pain-relief herbs and herbal formulas are best taken between meals.

Rule 8: The effectiveness of an herb depends on a variety of factors, including proper dose, health status of the person, product quality, and purity.

Rule 9: When purchasing herbs, keep in mind that the best values may be in herb shops or health food stores, but be careful about purity.

Rule 10: Fresh herbs and dried herbs have near-equal advantages when purity is not in question.

Bibliography

Heinerman, J. (1996). *Heinerman's encyclopedia of healing herbs and spices.* New York: Reward Books.

Note. From "The Ten Cardinal Rules of Herb Use," by G.M. Decker, 2006, *Clinical Journal of Oncology Nursing, 10*(2), p. 279. Copyright 2006 by Oncology Nursing Society. Reprinted with permission.

Resources for Reliable Information

Agency for Healthcare Research and Quality
- Cancer Prevention: Vitamin Supplements (www.ahrq.gov/clinic/uspstf/uspsvita.htm)
- Meditation Practices for Health: State of the Research (www.ahrq.gov/downloads/pub/evidence/pdf/meditation/medit.pdf)
- Melatonin: Sleep Disorders (www.ahrq.gov/news/press/pr2004/melatnpr.htm)

American Botanical Council
- Commission E Monographs (http://cms.herbalgram.org/commissione/index.html)
- HerbClip™ Online (http://cms.herbalgram.org/herbclip/index.html)
- HerbMedPro (membership fee) (http://cms.herbalgram.org/herbmedpro/overview.html)
- Monographs (http://abc.herbalgram.org/site/PageServer?pagename=Monographs)

American Cancer Society
- Complementary and Alternative Therapies (www.cancer.org/docroot/ETO/ETO_5.asp?sitearea=ETO)
- Nutrition for Children With Cancer (www.cancer.org/docroot/MBC/MBC_6_1_nutrition_for_children_with_cancer.asp)
- Nutrition for the Person with Cancer (www.cancer.org/docroot/MBC/MBC_6.asp?sitearea=ETO)

Institute of Medicine of the National Academies
- Summit on Integrative Medicine and the Health of the Public (www.iom.edu/en/Activities/Quality/IntegrativeMed/2009-FEB-25.aspx)

Selected Cancer Centers With Integrative Programs
- Arizona Center for Integrative Medicine (http://integrativemedicine.arizona.edu)
- Duke Integrative Medicine (www.dukeintegrativemedicine.org)
- George Washington Center for Integrative Medicine (www.integrativemedicinedc.com)

- Integrative Medicine Service at Memorial Sloan-Kettering Cancer Center (www.mskcc.org/mskcc/html/1979.cfm)
- Johns Hopkins Center for Complementary and Alternative Medicine (www .hopkinsmedicine.org/CAM)
- Osher Clinical Center for Complementary and Integrative Medical Therapies (www.brighamandwomens.org/medicine/oshercenter)
- Rosenthal Center for Complementary and Alternative Medicine (www .rosenthal.hs.columbia.edu)
- Stanford Center for Integrative Medicine: Clinical Services for Mind and Body (http://stanfordhospital.org/clinicsmedServices/clinics/complementary Medicine)
- University of Pittsburgh Center for Integrative Medicine (www.upmc.com/ Services/integrative-medicine/Pages/default.aspx)
- University of Texas M.D. Anderson Cancer Center Complementary/Integrative Medicine Education Resources (www.mdanderson.org/education -and-research/resources-for-professionals/clinical-tools-and-resources/ cimer/index.html)
- Vanderbilt Center for Integrative Medicine (www.vanderbilthealth.com/ integrativehealth)

Selected Journals
- *Advances in Mind-Body Medicine*
- *Alternative and Complementary Therapies*
- *Alternative Medicine Review*
- *Alternative Therapies in Health and Medicine*
- *BMC Complementary and Alternative Medicine*
- *Complementary Therapies in Clinical Practice*
- *Complementary Therapies in Medicine*
- *Evidence-Based Complementary and Alternative Medicine*
- *Focus on Alternative and Complementary Therapies*
- *HerbalGram: The Journal of the American Botanical Council*
- *Integrative Medicine: A Clinician's Journal*
- *Journal of Bodywork and Movement Therapies*
- *The Journal of Chinese Medicine*
- *The Journal of Alternative and Complementary Medicine*

U.S. Department of Agriculture
- Food and Nutrition Information Center (http://fnic.nal.usda.gov/nal_ display/index.php?tax_level=1&info_center=4)

U.S. Department of Health and Human Services
- White House Commission on Complementary and Alternative Medicine Policy (www.whccamp.hhs.gov/finalreport.html)

U.S. Federal Trade Commission
- Consumer Education on Diet, Health, and Fitness (www.ftc.gov/bcp/ menus/consumer/health.shtm)
- Operation False Cure (www.ftc.gov/bcp/edu/microsites/curious/share .shtml)

U.S. Food and Drug Administration
- Buying Medicines and Medical Products Online (www.fda.gov/For Consumers/ProtectYourSelf/default.htm)
- Center for Food Safety and Applied Nutrition: Dietary Supplements (www .fda.gov/Food/DietarySupplements/default.htm)
- Tips for Older Dietary Supplement Users (http://www.fda.gov/Food/ DietarySupplements/ConsumerInformation/ucm110493.htm)
- Tips for the Savvy Supplement User: Making Informed Decisions and Evaluating Information (www.fda.gov/Food/DietarySupplements/Consumer Information/ucm110567.htm)

U.S. National Institutes of Health (NIH)
- National Institute on Aging (www.nia.nih.gov)
- NIH SeniorHealth (http://nihseniorhealth.gov)
- National Institute of Arthritis and Musculoskeletal and Skin Diseases: Phytoestrogens and Bone Health (www.niams.nih.gov/Health_Info/Bone/ Osteoporosis/Menopause/default.asp)
- National Library of Medicine (www.nlm.nih.gov)
  - CAM on PubMed® (http://nccam.nih.gov/research/camonpubmed)
  - DIRLINE (http://dirline.nlm.nih.gov)
  - Dietary Supplements Labels Database (http://dietarysupplements.nlm .nih.gov/dietary)
  - MedlinePlus Drugs, Supplements and Herbal Information (www.nlm .nih.gov/medlineplus/druginformation.html)
  - MedlinePlus Complementary and Alternative Medicine Page (www.nlm .nih.gov/medlineplus/complementaryandalternativemedicine.html)
  - MedlinePlus Herbal Medicine Page (www.nlm.nih.gov/medlineplus/ herbalmedicine.html)
  - NLM FAQs: Dietary Supplements, Complementary or Alternative Medicines (www.nlm.nih.gov/services/dietsup.html)
- National Cancer Institute (NCI) (www.cancer.gov)
  - Cancer Information Service (http://cis.nci.nih.gov)
  - Office of Cancer Complementary and Alternative Medicine (OCCAM) (www.cancer.gov/cam)
  - NCI Fact Sheets (www.nci.nih.gov/cancertopics/factsheet)
    * Antioxidants and Cancer Prevention
    * Calcium and Cancer Prevention
    * Garlic and Cancer Prevention
    * Hyperthermia

  * Marijuana Use in Supportive Care for Cancer Patients
  * Mind-Body Medicine Practice in CAM
  * Physical Activity and Cancer
  * Red Wine and Cancer Prevention
  * Selenium and Vitamin E Cancer Prevention Trial (SELECT)
  * Tea and Cancer Prevention
- NCI PDQ® Cancer Information Summaries: Complementary and Alternative Medicine (www.cancer.gov/cancertopics/pdq/cam)
  * Acupuncture
  * Antineoplastons
  * Aromatherapy and Essential Oils
  * Cancell/Cantron/Protocel
  * Cartilage (bovine and shark)
  * Coenzyme Q10
  * Essiac/Flor-Essence
  * Gerson Therapy
  * Gonzalez Regimen
  * Hydrazine Sulfate
  * Laetrile/Amygdalin
  * Milk Thistle
  * Mistletoe Extract
  * Newcastle Disease Virus
  * PC-SPES
  * Selected Vegetables/Sun's Soup
  * Spirituality in Cancer Care
- National Cancer Institute PDQ® Cancer Information Summaries: Supportive and Palliative Care (Coping With Cancer) (www.cancer.gov/cancertopics/pdq/supportivecare)
  * Anxiety Disorder
  * Bereavement, Mourning, and Grief
  * Cardiopulmonary Symptoms
  * Cognitive Disorders and Delirium
  * Communication in Cancer Care
  * Depression
  * Fatigue
  * Fever, Sweats, and Hot Flashes
  * Gastrointestinal Complications
  * Hypercalcemia
  * Last Days of Life
  * Lymphedema
  * Nausea and Vomiting
  * Normal Adjustment and Distress
  * Nutrition in Cancer Care
  * Oral Complications of Chemotherapy and Head/Neck Radiation
  * Pain

* Pediatric Supportive Care
* Post-Traumatic Stress Disorder
* Pruritus
* Sexuality and Reproductive Issues
* Sleep Disorders
* Smoking Cessation and Continued Risk in Cancer Patients
* Spirituality in Cancer Care
* Substance Abuse Issues in Cancer
* Transitional Care Planning
– National Center for Complementary and Alternative Medicine (NCCAM) (General) (http://nccam.nih.gov/health)
– NCCAM Backgrounders (http://nccam.nih.gov/health/atoz.htm)
   * Acupuncture
   * Ayurvedic Medicine: An Introduction
   * Colloidal Silver Products
   * Energy Medicine
   * Manipulative and Body-Based Practices: An Overview
   * Massage Therapy as CAM
   * Meditation: An Introduction
   * Mind-Body Medicine: An Overview
   * Naturopathy: An Introduction
   * Reiki: An Introduction
   * Tai Chi for Health Purposes
   * Whole Medical Systems: An Overview
   * Yoga for Health: An Introduction
– NCCAM Herbs at a Glance (http://nccam.nih.gov/health/herbsat aglance.htm)
   * Aloe vera
   * Astralagus
   * Bilberry
   * Bitter orange
   * Black cohosh
   * Cat's claw
   * Chamomile
   * Chasteberry
   * Cranberry
   * Dandelion
   * Echinacea
   * Ephedra
   * European elder
   * Evening primrose oil
   * Fenugreek
   * Feverfew
   * Flaxseed and flaxseed oil
   * Garlic

* Ginger
* Ginkgo
* Ginseng (Asian)
* Goldenseal
* Grape seed extract
* Green tea
* Hawthorn
* Hoodia
* Horse chestnut
* Kava
* Lavender
* Licorice root
* Milk thistle
* Mistletoe (European)
* Noni
* Peppermint oil
* Red clover
* Saw palmetto
* Soy
* St. John's wort
* Thunder god vine
* Turmeric
* Valerian
* Yohimbe
– Office of Dietary Supplements Fact Sheets and Background Information (http://ods.od.nih.gov/Health_Information/Information_About_Individual_Dietary_Supplements.aspx)
  * Black cohosh
  * Botanical dietary supplements
  * Dietary supplements
  * Selenium
  * Vitamin A
  * Vitamin D
  * Vitamin E
– Office of Dietary Supplements (General) (http://ods.od.nih.gov/index.aspx)
  * Annual Bibliographies of Significant Advances in Dietary Supplement Research (http://ods.od.nih.gov/Research/Annual_Bibliographies.aspx)
  * Botanical Dietary Supplements: Background Information (http://ods.od.nih.gov/factsheets/botanicalbackground.asp)
  * Computer Access to Research on Dietary Supplements (CARDS) Database (http://ods.od.nih.gov/Research/CARDS_Database.aspx)
  * Dietary Supplement Ingredient Database (http://dietarysupplement database.usda.nih.gov)

* Frequently Asked Questions (http://ods.od.nih.gov/Health_Information/ODS_Frequently_Asked_Questions.aspx)
* International Bibliographic Information on Dietary Supplements Database (http://ods.od.nih.gov/Health_Information/IBIDS.aspx)
* NIH Botanical Research Centers Program (http://ods.od.nih.gov/Research/Dietary_Supplement_Research_Centers.aspx)

Science.gov
• Health and Medicine (www.science.gov/browse/w_127.htm)

Substance Abuse and Mental Health Services Administration
• Alternative Approaches to Mental Health Care (http://mentalhealth.samhsa.gov/publications/allpubs/KEN98-0044/default.asp)

World Health Organization (WHO)
• *WHO Strategy for Traditional Medicine, 2002–2005* (http://whqlibdoc.who.int/hq/2002/who_edm_trm_2002.1.pdf)
• *Guidelines on Developing Information on Proper Use of Traditional, Complementary, and Alternative Medicine* (http://apps.who.int/medicinedocs/en/d/Js5525e)

Index

U

University of Pittsburgh Center for Integrative Medicine, 176
University of Texas M.D. Anderson Cancer Center, Complementary/Integrative Medicine Education Resources, 176
unproven therapy, 160
U.S. Department of Agriculture, 176
U.S. Department of Health and Human Services, 176
U.S. Federal Trade Commission, 177
U.S. Food and Drug Administration, 153–154, 158, 177
U.S. National Institutes of Health (NIH), 153, 177–181

V

vaginal atrophy/thinning, 136
vaginal discharge, 133, 135*t*
vaginal dryness, 133, 135*t*
vaginismus, 133, 135*t*
valerian, 58*t*
    for anxiety, 79
    interactions with, 59*t*, 62*t*, 67*f*
    for menopausal symptoms, 106, 108
    sedation from, 46*f*
    for sleep-wake disturbances, 112
Vanderbilt Center for Integrative Medicine, 176
venlafaxine, for menopausal symptoms, 106
vitamin A
    for anemia, 120–121
    for anorexia-cachexia syndrome, 74
vitamin B$_2$, for depression, 93
vitamin B$_6$
    for anemia, 120
    for depression, 93
    for menopausal symptoms, 108
vitamin B$_{12}$, for anemia, 120–121
vitamin C, high-dose
    cancer growth/recurrence from, 50*t*
    interactions with, 67*f*
vitamin D
    for depression, 93
    for pain, 129
vitamin E
    for anemia, 120
    for menopausal symptoms, 106
vitamin supplements, for anorexia-cachexia syndrome, 74
vomiting, 123. *See also* nausea/vomiting

W

warfarin, interactions with, 61*t*–62*t*
Web site resources, 175–181
white horehound, for pain, 129
White House Commission on Complementary and Alternative Medicine Policy, 2, 176
wild carrot, sedation from, 46*f*
wild willow, clotting mechanisms affected by, 45*f*
wild yam
    cancer growth/recurrence from, 50*t*
    interactions with, 67*f*
    for menopausal symptoms, 106, 108
willow bark, interactions with, 59*t*
witch hazel, for menopausal symptoms, 108
withania root, sedation from, 46*f*
World Health Organization (WHO), 181

X

xerostomia, 145–147

Y

yerba mansa, sedation from, 46*f*
yerba santa, for xerostomia, 146
yew, interactions with, 65*t*
yoga
    for anxiety, 78
    certification/licensure for, 23*t*
    for depression, 92
    efficacy/safety of, 28*t*, 31*t*
    for fatigue, 102
    for menopausal symptoms, 107
    for pain, 129
    for sexual dysfunction, 136
Yoga Alliance, 23*t*
yohimbe
    interactions with, 59*t*, 62*t*, 64*t*
    for sexual dysfunction, 136
    for xerostomia, 146

Z

zinc
    for diarrhea, 98
    for menopausal symptoms, 108
    for taste change, 142
zone therapy. *See* reflexology